Signed First Edition

Love Izzy ♡

IZZY JUDD

January 2020

MICHAEL JOSEPH
an imprint of
PENGUIN BOOKS

mindfulness for mums

Simple ways to help you and your family feel calm, connected and content

Izzy Judd is a classically trained musician and her album with the electric string quartet Escala reached the top ten UK chart. Izzy married Harry Judd, a member of Mcfly, in 2012, and they have two children together. She has since been inspired to write about her experiences of motherhood, and *Dare to Dream* was her personal account of fertility struggles, IVF and miscarriage.

mindfulness
for Mums

Simple ways to help you and your family
feel calm, connected and content

IZZY JUDD

MICHAEL JOSEPH
an imprint of
PENGUIN BOOKS

MICHAEL JOSEPH

UK | USA | Canada | Ireland | Australia
India | New Zealand | South Africa

Michael Joseph is part of the Penguin Random House group of companies
whose addresses can be found at global.penguinrandomhouse.com

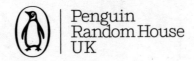

First published 2020
001

Copyright © Izzy Judd, 2020

Book, part and chapter title lettering by Letters by Julia
Heart illustrations by Alex Muravev

The moral right of the author has been asserted

Set in Garamond 13.5/16 pt Garamond MT Std
Typeset by Penguin Books
Printed in Great Britain by Clays Ltd, Elcograf S.p.A.

A CIP catalogue record for this book is available from the British Library

ISBN: 978–0–241–41122–3

www.greenpenguin.co.uk

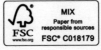

MIX
Paper from
responsible sources
FSC® C018179

Penguin Random House is committed to a
sustainable future for our business, our readers
and our planet. This book is made from Forest
Stewardship Council® certified paper.

For all the mums, especially mine.

Mindfulness:

'A mental state achieved by focusing one's awareness on the present moment, while calmly acknowledging and accepting one's feelings, thoughts and bodily sensations, used as a therapeutic technique.'

Contents

Why mindfulness?   I

Becoming mindful

How to bring mindfulness
into your day   15

My mindfulness corner   21

Mindful breathing cycle   25

One-minute mindfulness   29

Five ways to start your day   35

Breathing exercises with children   41

Just be

How to feel more grounded when
your head is in the clouds   49

Calm begins with me   53

Take five   57

5 4 3 2 1   63

WAIT and THINK   67

Nothing time   71

RAIN   77

Letting go   83

Go to bed, little one   91

May you be   103

Self-care

Let's talk about self-care   111

Looking after yourself in
the early days of motherhood   121

Contents

Sleep   133

Water   139

Chakras   143

Going outside

The weather and emotions   161

Nature   171

Simple ways to ease busy lives

Reduce the noise   179

Multitasking   189

Autopilot awareness   193

Perspective in motherhood   197

Slowing down   201

Truly listening   205

Spread a little happiness

Sharing mindful moments
with your family   213

Family list   229

Kindness   233

Charge up your hearts   243

Gratitude   247

A final thought . . .   261

Acknowledgements   263

Index   265

Why Mindfulness?

As mums we can find it difficult to be present; life is busier than ever and the challenges can at times feel overwhelming. You often hear 'Enjoy it – it goes so fast,' but some days when I'm finding this really hard I'm thinking, how?

We constantly question if we're doing a good enough job. Our mind is spinning with the mental load, not only emotionally but also practically. Our phones are beeping, mum guilt hangs over us and the daily noise of demands and expectations often means that our own well-being is overlooked, or we don't count it as being important enough on the never-ending to-do list.

I started to think about what I'm looking for as a

mum to find the calm. How can I ease frustration and stay patient when I feel I'm being tested? How do I let go of the need to be in control? How can I remember to be compassionate and to ask myself what I need right now for my own well-being? How can I nourish myself and accept the importance of self-care without feeling guilty or thinking it's indulgent to have time for me? How can I better communicate the way I'm feeling, to my family, my friends and to myself?

I grew up in a musical family, and my childhood was filled with love. I was mostly happy and confident, and yet ever since I can remember I have experienced anxiety. I believe my anxiety has always been part of who I am. Of course, as a young girl, I didn't understand it had a name; all I knew was that bedtime was scary. There wasn't a trigger, but I've always had a vivid imagination.

I dreaded bedtime; not because I was afraid of the dark – I just didn't want to be alone in my bedroom. I would often fall asleep OK, but then would wake up in what I now understand to be a panic. The sensation of fear was so strong it felt like I was running away from danger, and I was too scared to close my eyes and try to get back to sleep. My heart would be racing, my legs would shake, and once I'd found the courage to get out of bed I would quickly move into my parents' bed where I felt safe. I didn't know how to communicate how I was feeling, but it felt real and was frightening.

When I was twelve years old my eldest brother, Rupert, suffered a serious brain injury in a car accident. Although he miraculously survived, all these years later the lasting effects of his injury continue to be devastating and challenging for us all as a family and most of all for Rupert. The enormity of our family tragedy felt like confirmation that there *was* a reason to worry. Life as I had known it had changed overnight and I felt completely out of control. Fear of change and being out of control were two of the biggest worries that have remained with me over the years.

My teenage years and the severity of Rupert's injury completely shifted my perspective on life and although I had to grow up quickly I hadn't caught up emotionally. I didn't feel like my worries were big enough in comparison to the daily challenges Rupert was facing, and I didn't want to add to my parents' concerns. In hindsight I should have had counselling, but it wasn't offered to me and things like that just weren't as accessible then. All the while I was continuing to live with anxiety, although I still didn't know it had a name. It was just my normal.

In my twenties my anxiety became so bad that I was unable to spend any time alone, living in a heightened state of fear 24/7. I was going through what should have been one of the most exciting times in my life when Escala, the electric string quartet I was a member of, reached the final of *Britain's Got Talent* before signing a record deal and performing all over the world. I tried all sorts of treatments, some of which helped ease my anxiety, which by then had been diagnosed – and given a name.

But I still felt there was more I needed to do to help me understand my anxiety and, as it seemed to be a huge part of who I was, perhaps even attempt to become friends with it. This was when I came across mindfulness after Google kindly pointed me in the direction of Jon Kabat-Zinn, creator of the Center for Mindfulness in Medicine, Health Care and Society at the University of Massachusetts Medical School.

But what is mindfulness? Mindfulness is simply noticing what is happening in this moment without trying to change anything. It is about accepting and acknowledging our thoughts, then letting them pass with an understanding that nothing stays the same.

The revelation that you could be taught to live in

the present was a light-bulb moment for me, and as I started to practise this theory daily the more everything started to make sense. I have learned to notice and pay attention to my thoughts without judging them and I continue to learn to let thoughts go before beginning to believe in them. I have been able to access a sense of calm even in my most challenging moments and to remind myself to have an awareness of whether fear is determining my decisions. I have learned how important it is to take time to breathe and I have begun to understand that the mind isn't meant to sit still. In fact, if we allow ourselves to simply sit with our mind without external distractions, our most creative thoughts often come to us. There always seems to be something we believe is more important to be doing or responding to, but giving ourselves the opportunity to listen to our chatty mind gives us the space to find some answers and be inspired by new ideas.

Over the years I've turned to mindfulness many times, usually during periods of uncertainty and change. It has been the most powerful tool I have used, not only for managing mental health but also during difficult times emotionally, such as during our fertility struggles and more recently for the challenges motherhood brings.

When Kit was eight weeks old he had a cold and a fever, and over the following two days his symptoms got worse and he developed a nasty cough. Instinctively I knew something wasn't right so I took him to the doctor's where he was diagnosed with bronchiolitis. I was told to keep an eye on him but within minutes of getting home Kit began really struggling for breath. It was the most frightening experience, especially as I was alone with both children and Harry was out of contact in media interviews. We sadly don't have any family that live close by, so I felt I had no other option than to phone for an ambulance. Within moments the paramedics were at my front door. Kit had been really sick, so I had stripped him down to his nappy. I was not able to think clearly at all and was in a complete state of panic, not able to function. While one paramedic was examining Kit, the other calmly directed me to pack a bag with clothes and nappies, milk and bottles, a snack for Lola, my phone charger, house keys and a blanket to wrap round Kit. The ambulance then arrived and, with Lola strapped into a seat in the back with us, Kit was linked up to oxygen. It was utterly terrifying. He was admitted to hospital and shortly after Harry arrived to collect Lola, who by this point was understandably over it with tiredness and hunger.

However anxious I felt over the days that followed, there was an overriding natural instinct of wanting to protect Kit and I felt I had no other option than to cope. With the help of the wonderful NHS nurses and doctors he began to improve. It was when we arrived home three days later that my panic attacks returned, and if the children woke in the night, I immediately expected the worst-case scenario. I felt I couldn't cope with taking care of them and I didn't want to be left alone with the responsibility.

Not knowing which way to turn, it was Harry who suggested I take a mindfulness course to help me get back on track. Mindfulness was something I had practised regularly before becoming a mum and during my pregnancies, but I'd somehow lost my way with it since Lola had been born, perhaps wondering how I could find the time. I soon realized that there were small ways to introduce mindful practice into my day and that I needed it more than ever, especially when the children woke in the night.

Nobody can prepare you for what becoming a mum really feels like, and from the moment this tiny person arrives in your world nothing feels the same again. Having gone through so much to conceive our daughter, Lola, I hadn't given the reality of motherhood enough thought. All the practical stuff, like preparing the nursery, washing clothes, choosing a pram, was covered, but I was completely underprepared for the impact motherhood would have on me emotionally and how I would adjust to such a huge change in my life.

This is where the heart of *Mindfulness for Mums* comes from. I wanted to learn about how I could enjoy time with my children without being distracted. How I could quieten my inner critic and switch from constantly doing to just being. I wanted to explore other options to help manage Lola's and Kit's meltdowns or the endless inability to share that means I don't end up shouting and then spending the rest of the day feeling like I've failed them. I wanted to be able to talk kindly not only to Harry and the children but also to myself, and I wanted stressful moments to feel more manageable.

As I write, Lola is three and Kit has just turned two. It is fair to say my patience is often tested to the absolute limit and it feels hard to find a rational perspective when the simplicity of putting on a pair of shoes, choosing clothes or brushing teeth equals a meltdown for determined little minds. I'm constantly questioning my ability – am I getting this right, should I be responding in a different way? – all while having to remind myself who's in charge and taking many deep breaths!

Learning to pick battles, trying to change the subject, thinking of a different way to respond . . . wow, parenting is a daily lesson in how to find the calm, all while trying to navigate little people's understanding of the world and their big emotions. As each month passes I'm realizing that it's OK not to always get it right. Every child is unique and I'm still learning how to be the best I can be for each of my children. There will be days when I go to bed and feel I got something wrong, but I'm learning to remember that tomorrow is a new day and a chance to try again. I'm holding on to the moments that I suddenly get an impromptu 'I love you, Mummy', a squeezy cuddle and a look in their eyes that they only share with you.

Having lived with anxiety from a young age, I wanted to learn more about how mindfulness could also support my children with their own emotional development. I want to teach them the skills to take care of their own mental well-being and I have been amazed to discover Lola beginning to use the exercises even as young as three without being prompted. I have witnessed at first hand the benefits mindfulness is having and continues to have on all the family and it also reminds us of the importance of paying attention to the needs of others.

Mindfulness isn't something that requires hours of your time, and I have found that if you practise a little mindfulness every day, you will see a change in your mood, a general sense of calm and clarity, as well as reduced symptoms of anxiety. There is plenty of important information out there about how to look after our health in terms of exercise and nutrition, but we also need to think about our minds, so using mindfulness is a helpful way to connect the mind with the body.

Mindfulness for Mums aims to help us navigate our way through the challenges that parenthood brings with simple, short and effective exercises.

Some of the exercises in this book are intended for you to practise on your own, to help you take some time out, and these are marked with a single heart. There are also many that can be practised with your children, and these are marked with two hearts. The exercises are designed to be easily introduced into your day to help find the calm in the chaos without feeling like it's another job to add to the to-do list!

Although I have written the exercises with my children's ages in mind), they can be adapted for children of any age. Some exercises, particularly those involving writing, may require a little more help from you when practised with younger children.

It is important to remember that we are all trying to do our best and are learning every day about how to manage our expectations and emotions. I know that as quickly as I can feel such love and compassion in motherhood, I can just as quickly feel impatient and frustrated. The exercises in this book are there to help guide and support; they are not something that you should feel like you've got right or wrong or which add to your mental load of what you think you should be doing for yourself and your children. Simply thinking of it as a little mindful practice a day will go a long way to help and if while reading the exercises you try something that doesn't work for you or your family that day, let it go and try again another day. You may find some exercises resonate with you more than others, so go with what feels right for you.

Motherhood is the greatest thing and the toughest thing all at once. I hope *Mindfulness for Mums* will support you and hold your hand through the challenging, exhausting and happy days, and that it's something you can share with your family over the years.

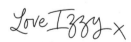

Becoming mindful

How to bring mindfulness into your day

♡

I want to begin this first exercise by asking you to think of a mindfulness affirmation. An affirmation is a short and powerful statement that if repeated often enough is something that can help overcome negative thoughts and encourage us to believe in ourselves with strength and positivity.

It is important you find an affirmation that feels right for you. Here are some suggestions:

- Let go.
- I am enough.

- Everything I need is within me.

- I matter.

- I am capable.

- May I be calm.

- All is well, all is calm, I am safe.

You can use this affirmation as a reminder to bring mindfulness into your day. It may change depending on your mood, but you might find one or two that resonate with you more than others. During any point in the day, when you feel overwhelmed or challenged, say this affirmation to yourself. These words will act as a trigger to acknowledge that you need to take a mindful pause.

What to do when you take a mindful pause:

- Ground your feet into the floor beneath you.

- Relax your shoulders and ease any tension you feel in the body.

- Notice the single task you are doing in that moment.

- Breathe in slowly for the count of four, pause for two, then breathe

out for the count of four. This can
be repeated as many times as you
need or for as long as you have!

- As you breathe, think or speak
  your affirmation; this could be
  once or as many times as needed.

It is then simply about finding pockets of time in
the day to allow your mind and body to pause, to
take a breath, focus yourself in the present and pay
attention to the task you are completing without
allowing your mind to become overloaded with all
the other jobs that need your attention. I promise
we all have moments to pause in the day; it's about
learning to find them!

When do I have time to practise mindfulness?

Hopefully you will discover through the exercises in
this book that the chance to be mindful is all around
us – we just need to open ourselves up to noticing
the opportunities. By taking time out to find these
little moments in the day, you will begin to notice
space in your mind for your thoughts to become
clearer, your body will feel calmer, your approach to

challenging situations will feel more manageable, you will be able to enjoy time with your loved ones and it will help to improve relationships – not only with others but also with yourself.

Here are some simple examples of when to take a mindful pause in the day:

- The moment your feet touch the ground in the morning.

- While waiting for the kettle to boil.

- Brushing your children's hair or your own.

- Moisturizing your face.

- Before pressing start on the washing machine.

- Putting on the children's shoes or your own.

- Starting up your phone or laptop.

- In the queue at the post office or shops.

- While cooking.

- During the children's bath time.

- When you close the children's
  bedroom door at night.

You might also find it helpful to use notes as a reminder to take a pause. For example, on top of your laptop, inside your purse or on your bedside table you can place a note saying 'Mindful pause', or write a note with a mindful affirmation such as 'Let go'. This is a gentle prompt to remember to pause, breathe and bring your attention to the present moment.

One example of where to bring your attention for a 'Mindful pause' is at your front door. This could be before leaving the house or arriving home. For me personally, in the morning when we finally get to the door to leave I can feel quite flustered, after a race against the clock and trying to think if I've remembered everything for the children (let alone myself!), I appreciate taking a 'Mindful pause' in this moment as I reach to turn the door handle. Equally, arriving home could be to either a quiet house or a hectic teatime, so by taking a 'Mindful pause' as your keys turn in the lock, this allows us a moment to find the right headspace for what is to follow in our day.

Something I have noticed that affects me more

and more in motherhood is the volume of noise, not only mentally from the busyness of my thoughts but also noise from the children. This can be anything from whinging to overexcitement or crying. Whatever the noise, I crave peace. Using this exercise can help find that space for quiet, allowing us not to be swept along with the noise and instead reminding us to release tension, frustration or impatience, and a chance to mentally check out of the chaos for a moment before stepping back in, hopefully with a sense of calm and clarity.

It is very important to remember that we don't always get it right; some days will always feel tougher than others. Don't be hard on yourself. There is always a chance to start again tomorrow, and hopefully by dipping in and out of this book for inspiration and guidance it will help you manage the challenging moments as well as being able to enjoy the happy ones!

My mindfulness corner

A mindfulness corner is a place that each member of the family understands is for quiet moments, where you have permission to sit peacefully. It is a space where I often practise mindful activities, but it is also a place I go to just be. Sometimes half the battle is making time to just sit down and not feel like you should be doing something else. Creating a space in your home where you and your family can practise mindfulness feeling safe, cosy and comfortable is a good place to start on your path to more mindful living.

To begin with you could have a think together about what you might like to have in your mindfulness corner and what would help you feel able to relax.

Here are some of the items we have chosen for our own:

- A sheepskin rug to comfort tired feet.
- A comfortable chair or cushion to rest on.
- Books/magazines.
- A blanket to snuggle up in.
- A diffuser to help us feel calmer; we call this fairy mist.
- A bell to signal the start and end of our mindful practice.

Initially I had my own mindfulness corner in the house and by seeing me there, practising mindfulness, everyone became inquisitive and would ask questions about what I was doing. Once I explained what the space was for I found the children naturally gravitated to the space too and joined me, often mirroring my behaviour. Involving them in the time I spent practising mindfulness was a natural progression.

You could also create a mindfulness corner in your child's bedroom. I have found it very helpful for Lola to have a calm place to go when she is overtired, becoming frustrated at having to share her toys with Kit, or even when we all just need a moment to step away from each other before a situation spirals. Kit is a little younger, but he also has his own space where we sit and read books to him so he can begin to understand that this is his quiet place.

I spoke to Lola about what she would like to have in her mindfulness corner. We placed a cushion next to a box containing her favourite blanket, and we have some books, a snow globe that is relaxing and focuses attention, a puzzle and some cuddly toys. Every few weeks we change the items in Lola's box to keep her inspired and interested.

I feel uncomfortable using phrases like 'the naughty step' and 'go to your room', but in those moments when we inevitably lose our temper it is tempting to shout them in desperation. There are many times as a mum I have wished I had handled things differently, so having a mindfulness corner has given me another option and one that I feel has had a more positive impact for everyone.

In those moments of chaos when you feel like no one is listening and voices are getting louder, I have found by offering a break in our mindful corner it gives my response to a challenging situation a different feel and enables me to not only step away from the situation but it also gives my children the opportunity to calm down and have space from one another too.

I hope you enjoy creating a peaceful corner in your home for you and your family.

Mindful breathing cycle

'Inhale love, exhale gratitude.'

Doing something as simple as relaxing and paying attention to your breathing can really help you feel calmer and more mindful.

You will feel the benefits of this exercise even if you have as little as one minute to sit and breathe. However, as you begin to practise more regularly, you might find you are able to extend the time for as long as you need (or have!).

Before you start, it is important that you feel comfortable, so these are some suggestions that I use to help with that, but you might find a way that suits you better.

To begin:

- Sit comfortably, resting your hands gently on your lap, and straighten your upper body.

- Let the soles of your feet ground themselves on the floor.

- Relax your shoulders downwards from your ears and lower your chin slightly.

- Allow your face to relax, paying attention to releasing any tension around your jaw and mouth and between your eyes.

- Lower your gaze or, if you would like to, slowly close your eyes.

- Relax and bring attention to the breath.

When you are comfortable you can begin a breathing cycle. *This is also a simple way to count the breath with your child:*

- Breathe in slowly for four counts.

- Pause for two counts.

Mindful breathing cycle

- Breathe out slowly for four counts.
  During the pause notice the stillness.

Counting the breath is a lovely way to slow down our breathing and quieten the mind.

You could try thinking of the word 'Let' as you inhale and 'Go' as you exhale. This can help release tension as you visualize it leaving your body along with the breath.

You might notice your mind wandering, with thoughts coming and going. There may also be certain times in the day that your mind is busier. Instead of trying to stop your thoughts, which will inevitably cause you to engage with them, without judgement bring your attention back to the breathing cycle.

When you are ready slowly open your eyes, or lift your gaze and take a moment to observe how your mind and body feel as you bring your attention back to the room.

Enjoy the moment of feeling stillness and peace.

One-minute mindfulness

♡

Knowing when and how to begin practising mindfulness isn't always easy. Often the biggest barrier to overcome, though, is time – most of us feel like we don't have enough time to do all the things that need doing, and mindfulness might not feel like a priority. Setting a reminder first thing in the morning or before bed is a great way to introduce a mindfulness routine into our day.

Even if we just practise for one minute, we can feel the benefits of giving ourselves permission to sit, pause and breathe. Setting our intention to practise a breathing cycle (see page 26) for one minute during our day seems a good way to start and we can extend the time as we feel more comfortable.

One minute is also a manageable amount of time for our children's attention.

Here are a few exercises you can try:

Checking in with mind, body, breath

Ask yourself these questions:

- How does my mind feel in this moment? *Busy, quiet, a little bit fuzzy.*

- How does my body feel in this moment? *Tired, energized or depleted.*

- How does my breath feel? *Is it high up in my chest, lower down in my tummy, long or short?*

First thing in the morning my mind can be full of thoughts. I feel a surge of adrenaline in my body and my breath is usually in my chest and quite short. It helps to familiarize ourselves with these sensations and not be fearful of them.

As you begin to practise this daily you may begin to notice a pattern. It reminds us to pay attention to our mind, body and breath throughout the day. There is no need to change anything; we are simply observing and checking in with ourselves.

Hear and feel

I find this exercise very helpful at bedtime when my imagination can become particularly active.

- Take a moment to listen to three sounds you can hear.

  For example, the buzz from a bathroom light, traffic noise outside, a clock ticking.

- Then notice three things you can feel.

  For example, the softness of your pillow, toes under the duvet cover, a warm breath through your nostrils as you exhale.

This helps to focus the mind in the present and prevents unwanted or anxious thoughts when trying to settle down for a restful night's sleep.

Body scan

This exercise can be done sitting or lying down.

- Whether you are sitting or lying, notice the weight of your body and the points where your body is grounded, such as your feet touching the floor.

- Begin with a few deep breaths.

- As you inhale feel the breath fill your body, and as you exhale enjoy the sensation of your body releasing tension and letting go.

- As you move up the body imagine each part of your body softening and relaxing.

- Starting with the feet, slowly move up to the legs, stomach, chest, arms, hands and face.

- You can go into more detail. For example, thinking of each finger/ different parts of the face.

- You might like to explore physically tensing each part of the body – scrunching up your toes or creating a fist with your hand, for example – on the inhale and releasing on the exhale.

- You can also tense all the body with the inhale, hold and then as you exhale release the tension.

The physical feeling of relaxation and letting go can help us to relax more deeply.

The important thing to remember with all these exercises is to use the ones that feel right for you and don't be afraid to adapt them to suit you. This is *your* mindful moment.

five ways to start your day ♡

Since becoming a mum, I soon realized that starting my day had a very new feeling to it. With young children there is no certainty about when the day might begin and there is also no gentle way of waking up. You're launched straight into the day and your children's needs inevitably come first.

This is something I found quite difficult to adjust to, not just physically but also mentally. Lack of sleep from unexpected wake-up calls and a surge of adrenaline on waking often contributed to a feeling of anxiety. I realized that I needed to address this and think of another way to begin my day. Of course, we can't always predict when our children's day will start, but we can try to get ahead of the game.

Once they were a little older and in a slightly more predictable routine I started to set my alarm thirty minutes before I expected Lola and Kit to wake up. This might seem obvious, but for me it was a revelation!

Of course, this isn't possible every morning and children are unpredictable; however, when I am able to have this time for myself I notice a shift in my mood. Even to have a few slower mornings and peaceful showers a week helps me to feel that some of my own well-being has been taken care of and therefore I feel better prepared for the day ahead. If you find the screen from your phone an instant distraction, you might want to think about replacing the alarm on your phone with an old-school alarm clock.

Another thing that I do to try to help myself feel like I've already achieved something at the start of the day is to prepare as much as I can for the morning routine the night before, so I'm not rushing around like a madwoman trying to get out of the door! For example, getting clothes ready for the children and myself, having an empty dishwasher and preparing food such as packed lunches.

Starting the day feeling organized and calm is so important to how the rest of my day goes, so with

36

that in mind I began to think about other ways to help me feel grounded first thing in the morning too.

I'm sharing five nurturing ways to start the day, which I hope you will also find beneficial. You might find other things that work for you too, but the important thing is to do things that make you feel positive and calmer at the beginning of the day.

1. Sit on the side of your bed and let your feet touch the ground. Take a moment to allow yourself to feel grounded to the earth. I love a sheepskin rug next to my bed as this is the first thing I feel in the morning, which is very comforting. Take a deep breath in and then, when breathing out, say the words 'I ground myself' either in your head or out loud.

2. Place one hand on your heart, this simple action alone is soothing.

3. Take a deep breath in and then, when breathing out, say the words 'Today I choose patience' either in your head or out loud. You can change the word 'patience' to anything that suits you in that moment, for example you could use

words like 'kindness' or 'forgiveness'. At this point you can introduce a one-minute mindful practice. This could be concentrating on a breathing cycle (see page 26), an exercise to check in with your mind, body and breath (see page 30), or a body scan (see page 32).

4. Carry out the extended mountain pose yoga exercise.

- Standing tall with your feet hip width apart, relax your shoulders down from the ears.

- With your hands resting by your sides raise them up with palms facing upwards, breathe in, bringing the hands up from the side in a large circle and placing them together above your head in the prayer position.

- Breathe out and bring your hands down from the prayer position with your palms facing down in a circle back down to your sides.

There are many benefits to practising mountain pose, including waking up every muscle in your body and helping to improve posture. Personally, it makes me feel empowered for the day ahead.

5. When filling up your children's water bottles, fill up a large bottle of water for yourself as a reminder to stay hydrated. There are many benefits to drinking water. Keeping hydrated can increase your energy, relieve fatigue, help improve complexion and boost the immune system. See also Water on page 139.

Hopefully finding five ways to start every day will help to give you a moment to energize and centre yourself for the day ahead and in return leave you feeling a little calmer and more grounded.

Breathing exercises with children

♡♡

Practising mindfulness from a young age helps to access an inner calm and the ability to understand when the mind and body are relaxed. It also assists with developing key skills such as concentration, focus, self-awareness, reasoning and discipline.

Children are most likely to follow by example so when possible practise and talk about mindfulness openly in front of your children. I have discovered that if I sit in our mindfulness corner and take one minute out of a busy day to breathe, Lola and Kit are intrigued by what I'm doing. I've prepared a box of quiet toys and books for them both to play with when they join me in the mindfulness corner, and I've been amazed that most of the time they sit still, understanding that this is quiet time. Lola has begun to copy my actions and sits next to me with her eyes closed and we all enjoy a moment of silence, which is always very welcome in our noisy house!

The key to practising mindfulness is learning to understand how to connect with the breath. Our breath is always there for us to use and plays a crucial role in calming down the nervous system.

We all know instinctively how to breathe, but as we grow older stress often changes the way we breathe and the breath tends to move higher up into the chest. We breathe quicker, meaning we take in less air, and therefore our bodies aren't getting enough oxygen to replenish our brain and other vital organs with essential nutrients.

If you watch a baby breathing, you see that they naturally breathe deeply from the abdomen. When Lola and Kit were babies, after a feed I would often lie them on me and focus on slowing down my breathing and imagine my tummy filling up with air like a balloon before releasing the breath slowly. I found this very soothing and I still use this as a way to calm Lola and Kit down if they are upset or fractious.

Mindful breathing

- Before practising mindful breathing with a child, begin by finding a peaceful place in your home; this could be your mindfulness corner.

- Find some comfortable chairs or cushions to sit on, or children can sit on your lap.

- Allow everyone a chance to settle; you could begin by reading a book to calm down and find some quiet and focus.

- Using a timer and a bell, set a short session of one minute. Children usually love to ring the bell at the start and end of each mindful breathing practice.

- During this time you can practise a mindful breathing cycle (see page 25). Invite your child to sit quietly with you.

Begin with one-minute sessions here and there throughout your week and as the children get used to this the length of time can be extended.

As they learn the breathing games below these can be practised together during these sessions.

Breathing games to share
with your children

• Teddy breathing

Lying down, ask your child to place a favourite teddy on their tummy; you can place a teddy on your tummy too.

Ask them to watch the teddy moving up and down with their breath. This isn't about changing anything or slowing down the breath; it is simply teaching us to notice and observe our breathing.

• Snake breathing

Ask your child to sit with their back straight.

With their hands on their tummy ask them to listen to your words.

'Breathe in for four seconds and feel your tummy fill up like a balloon.'

'As you breathe out make the sound of a snake hissing for as long as you can while I count to eight.'

Repeat this exercise as many times as you like.

• Breathing hands

This is a very gentle exercise. Sit your child in front of you facing away from you and encourage them to breathe with you.

Explain that you will take three deep breaths together while you place your hands on their back, shoulders and head.

Say the words 'Breathe in slowly, breathe out slowly'. Then take three deep breaths in and out with your hands on their back, three deep breaths in and out with your hands on their shoulders, and three deep breaths in and out with your hands on their head.

Lola likes to swap positions and do the same for me. This encourages us both to slow down. I have used this technique when Lola is overtired and we can both feel quite irritable – usually at the end of the day!

• Bath time

Water is naturally relaxing – you can add a little lavender to the water and invite your child to lie down and watch the water rise and fall on their tummies as they breathe in and out.

Encourage your child to breathe in for four counts, hold for two counts, then breathe out for four.

This is a gentle way to wind down and prepare children for a good night's sleep.

Just be

How to feel more grounded when your head is in the clouds ♡

There are days when it might feel like we are emotionally, mentally and physically being thrown all over the place. When we are unsupported it is very easy to end up feeling off balance and vulnerable. I know as a mum there have been many occasions when I have felt like I'm floating, trying to grasp and manage so many aspects of motherhood. The mental load quickly piles up with everything that needs to be done, so this exercise can help to bring my awareness back down to earth.

If we spend too much time thinking and worrying, we can get caught up with the story we are creating and imagining. It is natural to daydream but too much overthinking can shift our attention further away from the reality of the situation.

For example, if Harry and I have a day out planned with the children, I go through all the worst-case scenarios in my mind and then when I get to the end of the day I wonder if I missed out on simply being able to enjoy the day with the children!

Practising a short grounding exercise regularly can bring us back to the moment we are in, no matter what might be going on around us. It is also a quick way to help when we are anxious or overwhelmed.

What does it mean to feel grounded? Very simply, to feel grounded is to be connected to the earth and remain present in mind and body. Roots are solid and give us a sense of stability. Visualizing the roots of a tree can help us feel planted when everything around us might seem unsteady.

Grounding exercise: My forest

With trees being such an obvious visual reference this is a great exercise to adapt and share with your children in times of worry or when little minds are feeling overwhelmed.

- You can practise this exercise standing, sitting or lying down and as always it is important that you feel comfortable.

- Standing or sitting, with your feet slightly apart, plant the soles of your feet into the floor beneath you. If you are lying down, it might help to raise your knees and plant your feet into the bed or floor.

- Take a moment to focus on grounding your feet into the earth before lowering your gaze or gently closing your eyes.

- Take a few deep mindful breaths, remembering to soften the muscles in your face and allowing your body and shoulders to relax.

- Once you are feeling settled imagine you are standing in a beautiful forest surrounded by tall strong trees. You can hear the wind rustling through the leaves, the birds are singing and you notice that every tree is a different shade of green. Now imagine you are one of these trees and begin to slowly visualize the roots of your tree growing down from your feet, deep into the earth. Even though your branches might be moving in the breeze and leaves rustling in the wind, you are able to remain solid, strong, tall and stable no matter what life might throw at you.

Like you now, your tree is grounded and safe. It might help to think the words 'I feel grounded, I feel strong, I feel safe'.

- You can stay in the forest for as long as you need, then when you are ready slowly open your eyes and focus your gaze back up into the room.

Calm begins with me

♡

'When little people are overwhelmed by big
emotions, it's our job to share our calm,
not to join their chaos.' – L. R. Knost

Calm Begins With Me is a practical exercise that works quickly and effectively and can be used in many different situations when we need to take a moment to gather our thoughts. It gives us the opportunity to pause and think about our reaction, especially when we are being challenged by our emotions.

I often find myself feeling consumed by the needs of my children, as I'm sure so many of us do. Simple daily tasks with Lola and Kit, such as a trip to the shops, waiting in a queue at the post office, meal times or choosing clothes to wear, can end up in a meltdown (usually from them, sometimes from me!), even after trying my best to manage the situation calmly.

It is tough to manage surges of emotion while our patience is being tested, especially as each small challenging moment starts to pile up throughout the day, affecting our overall mood, which can end up with us feeling drained and exhausted!

I have found Calm Begins With Me a useful tool to use as a reminder that our energy and words can impact on those around us and change how they might react to a situation, something I certainly find with the children, who tend to mirror my behaviour and moods. This is a beneficial exercise to use at home with the family, but it also translates when out and about or at work. It is very effective in times of need when you might feel anxious, under pressure, frustrated or tense and in need of a reminder that you have the power to cope and to respond in the way you would like to.

This is how Calm Begins With Me works:

- Start by touching your thumb with your first finger, then your thumb with your second finger continuing with third and fourth fingers.

- Each time you press a finger with your thumb say these words:

  First finger – 'calm'.
  Second finger – 'begins'.
  Third finger – 'with'.
  Fourth finger – 'me'.

- The word 'calm' can be replaced with any word you might need for the situation or mood you are in. For example, 'compassion', 'patience', 'love', 'kindness'.

  You can practise this action with both hands at the same time and repeat the phrase as many times as you need. I say the phrase up to four times.

If you practise this regularly, you'll find that the simple physical action is a good trigger to bring you back to a sense of calm, which in turn will hopefully encourage others to do the same.

Take five

It is important to remind ourselves to take time out in our day to simply breathe. Focusing on just counting your breath offers a mindful way to bring your awareness into the present moment.

Breathing isn't just necessary for life. Deep breathing is one of the best things you can do for your overall health. It:

- Rests and regenerates mind and body.
- Strengthens the immune system.
- Improves digestion.
- Has long-term benefits for physical health.

- Benefits our hormonal system, including stress hormones.

- Allows peace and stillness.

- Focuses our attention.

- Taking time for five mindful breaths gives the mind and body a chance to slow down and relax.

- Breathing helps children to develop concentration as well as an understanding of mindfulness.

Take five gives us the chance to practise slow mindful breathing. It can be used any time, anywhere and can be practised with the family. As a visual and sensory exercise children respond well to it and have found it a useful tool at school as it can easily be practised at their desk when they need a moment to calm down or to focus their attention.

What I love about this exercise is that it can stay with a child for their lifetime. It can be practised with your eyes open or closed. Some people find it easier to focus on the breath with their eyes closed, whereas others like to watch the visual action to help focus the mind on the breath.

- Place your hand in front of you with your palm facing away from you.

- Spread your fingers wide.

- Keep the first finger of your other hand on the skin while you trace the outline of your hand slowly.

- Begin by moving your first finger up the side of your thumb while breathing in.

- When you breathe, breathe deeply from your stomach rather than taking shallow breaths from higher up in your chest. It is important to breathe from your stomach to get sufficient oxygen into the blood, which supplies energy to your muscles and organs. Taking slow, deep breaths like this also slows you down.

- As you breathe out move your first finger down the other side of your thumb.

- Repeat this action with your first, second, third and fourth fingers, each time breathing in as you trace up the

side of your finger and breathing out
as you trace back down the other side
of your finger.

- This enables us to take five slow deep
breaths.

- If you would like to continue and take
five more breaths, you can repeat the
action backwards from your fourth
finger back to your thumb.

Another way to teach your child this exercise is to
each place one hand on each other's, so that your
palms are touching and fingers aligned, then with
your spare hand, together you can trace up and down
the fingers to help slow down your child's breathing
as you take five breaths. The soothing touch will
connect, calm and bring the two of you. Lola likes to
call this star-print breathing, which I love.

Just focusing on your five breaths will help you
feel more peaceful and grounded, but you might
also like to think of these things:

- Notice how the breath moves in
the body.

- Really pay attention to tracing your hand slowly. This gives the breath a chance to slow down.

- While breathing imagine a colour or image that makes you feel calm and happy.

- Visualize a golden balloon in your stomach expanding as you breathe in and releasing as you breathe out. This will encourage you to breathe from your stomach rather than your chest.

- Pay attention to the sound of your breathing and observe the mind and body relaxing as you practise.

5 4 3 2 1

'Never hurry, never worry, and don't
forget to smell the flowers along the way.'

Taking time to look at life through our children's eyes and discover our senses as if for the first time is one of the best ways to practise mindfulness on a daily basis, and it doesn't require us to find extra time in our already busy day.

I've learned that Lola and Kit rarely think about the past or the future, and so children are our greatest teachers in bringing us back to the present, rather than reliving our past or imagining our future. Paying attention to what we can see, hear, touch, smell and taste helps us take in the present moment. This is a lovely exercise to share with the family and allows us to spend time observing the simple joys that can go unnoticed each day. Not only does this benefit us, it will also start teaching our children to be mindful and help them to expand their own awareness.

This exercise has traditionally been used to calm anxiety during extreme times of worry. Bringing our attention to the senses helps ground us and by counting what you become aware of it can shift our focus to our immediate surroundings and therefore hopefully interrupt the spinning of our thoughts.

You simply look for . . .

- Five things you can see.

  Door, mug, book, window, candle.

- Four things you can hear.

  Clock ticking, phone ringing, people talking, traffic.

- Three things you can touch.

  Table, hands, chair.

- Two things you can smell.

  Cut grass, perfume.

- One thing you can taste.

Coffee.

As you become more settled into the exercise you will discover how detailed you can become with your senses. For example, you might go into more detail about the colour of the mug, the volume of the phone ringing, the texture of the chair, the undertones to the scent of the perfume and the aftertaste of a coffee.

When I do this with Lola I love the fact that we take time together to observe the simple joys that surround us and at the same time introduce some mindfulness into our days.

I use Lola's answers to ask questions about the things that she notices and then together we observe our surroundings in greater detail. It's a really lovely way to have a conversation too. Lola might answer like this:

- What we can see: the ducks swimming in the pond.

- What we can hear: the birds in our garden (mixed in with the sound of aeroplanes!).

- What we can touch: the fur on our cat.

- What we can smell: stopping to smell the flowers on a walk to the park.

- What we can taste: something yummy like Lola's favourite banana milkshake!

Our conversation will build so that soon we are talking in more detail about the colour of the pond and what else is in there, we'll discuss whether the birds are loud or quiet, what the fur feels like, whether the flowers smell sweet and whether our milkshake has enough banana in it! I've learned that each time we practise this exercise we can become more creative and we often give unexpected or very detailed answers to surprise one another.

WAIT and THINK

♡

'May I speak truthfully and with kindness.'

I know that when I'm tired, hungry, haven't stopped all day or had a long night with disturbed sleep, the first person I'm likely to snap at is Harry and I don't even mean half the things I say! The people closest to us are usually the ones we take things out on and often all too quickly and easily. Life is busy and there can be little time left in the day for each other, let alone for yourself. Trying to strike a balance between the juggle of work and family life is something I know so many of us can relate to. Snatching conversations here and there while also trying to look after tiny humans can be a daily challenge!

WAIT is an exercise that can be used in many situations, not only at home with the family but also at work or with friends. It reminds us to check when is the right time to talk – which perhaps during a toddler meltdown might not be the optimum moment! – and when to wait.

Since I started using WAIT, it has stopped me from saying things that I know I would regret.

How to use the acronym WAIT

Before responding to something in the heat of the moment ask yourself:

Why

Am

I

Talking?

In a difficult moment thinking 'WAIT' gives us a chance to stop and think before we speak. It encourages healthy communication with one another and helps us stay connected and rational.

When using the exercise, during your moment's pause it can be uscful to think of another acronym called THINK.

Is what I'm about to say:

> **T**rue? Check the accuracy in your words.
>
> **H**elpful? Is what I am about to say helpful to myself and others?
>
> **I**nspiring? Will my words inspire?
>
> **N**ecessary? Am I being constructive?
>
> **K**ind? I must try to be kind with the words I speak.

As children we hear the expression 'Think before you speak', but as adults we can forget to practise this. THINK not only helps remind us of this but also teaches our children to take a step back and pause, encouraging kinder and more effective communication.

Most importantly using WAIT and THINK gives us the chance and space to question how we really feel and if and how we would like to respond.

- Think before you speak.
- Am I saying this from a place of anger?
- Am I being respectful?
- Could my words be misinterpreted?
- Am I being kind not only to others but also to myself?

Nothing time

♡

'Life is what happens to you when you're
busy making other plans.' – John Lennon

I have never been very good at doing nothing. I'd
even go as far as to say that sitting with my thoughts
has at times felt uncomfortable and overwhelming.
Keeping busy quickly became a method to avoid
anxiety. Over time I've come to understand how
vital doing nothing is when it comes to looking after
the health of my mind. I have a tendency during
periods of stress or worry to keep as busy as possible, not wanting to let go in fear of losing control.
However, letting go of being in control is exactly
what *is* needed. When I stop allowing myself the
chance to sit and do nothing it sets off alarm bells

that something might not be quite right. In order to release anxiety it is key to allow yourself to let go.

Studies show that people are generally happier and more relaxed on the weekends, which makes sense. We can choose our own activities and the pace of life slows down. There is usually less responsibility and fewer things to do than during the week and we are more likely to have family and friends around us or spend longer in our PJs!

Being too busy can be counterproductive and as a result we often become more exhausted, stressed and overstimulated. We're told that babies who are overstimulated find it harder to sleep, so why should that be any different for adults?

The ability to do nothing is crucial for our well-being, especially to give our brain and body a chance to rest. It is in the stillness and during quieter moments that we can be our most creative and inspired selves. If we are constantly busy, we don't give ourselves the space to stop and recharge our batteries.

Simply being is something I continue to work on with the help of mindfulness. The first step is giving yourself permission to just be with no guilt attached to it. I find it helpful to allocate time where I don't have to achieve or do anything, even for five minutes. In this time I enjoy getting into comfy clothes and being on the sofa, either listening to the radio or reading a magazine. I also find it helpful to sit outside and take some mindful breaths; the sound of nature is peaceful, and fresh air is just as important for us as it is our children. Taking a moment to pause helps us to unwind into nothing. Whatever your nothing time looks like, indulge in it and allow yourself the time.

Nothing time for children

We are role models to our children, so if they observe us constantly busy they will copy. As a parent I know at times I have found it a pressure to fill Lola and Kit's time with an activity, feeling like we've had an unproductive day if we have simply stayed at home. If I hear Lola say the words 'I'm bored', I'm now learning to embrace it rather than thinking it means that I'm not doing enough to stimulate or entertain her. It's important for children to learn how to do nothing and a good reminder for us too. Children need nothing time just as much as we do to relax and unwind. It is while doing nothing that they have the chance to be creative and curious while exploring their surroundings and learning more about themselves. It encourages them to daydream and be reflective, which can help emotional development.

These days there are more toys available than ever, so I know I can forget how to be imaginative with play time. If we strip the toys back, I find I'm able to engage in role play and be swept along with the beauty and innocence of a child's imagination. Playtime for adults is a great way to remember what it's like to have fun like a child again and remember the simple joys of being young. I'm sure if you let go enough it will release those happy endorphins!

Boredom jar

I've decided that when Lola or Kit inevitably tell me they're bored in the years to come, I'm going to say that's exciting because now you can go and be imaginative!

The boredom jar is a fun exercise to encourage children to start thinking creatively about new activities they can do. This can be a very helpful go-to during school holidays!

All they need to do is write a list of activities and

place them in the jar, then each day they can take out an activity to complete.

- Make up a play.
- Make a gift for a friend.
- Build a den.
- Write a letter and post it.
- Have a teddy bears' picnic.
- Choose some clothes and toys that you don't use any more to take to the charity shop.
- Build something out of Lego.
- Play with a toy you haven't played with in a while.
- Bake cookies with Mum or Dad.
- Go to the library to choose some new books.
- Make something from a box.
- Help wash the car.
- Play a board game.
- Make up a story.

- Plant some flowers.
- Help tidy your bedroom.
- The memory game. (Choose ten items or more and place them on a tray, then memorize them before covering with a tea towel. Then recite the items you can remember.)
- Make a memory box from a shoebox.

RAIN

As mums we go through all sorts of emotions during a day. We are not only managing our own emotions but also those of our family. These emotions, piled on top of each other, can enhance a situation that on its own might feel more manageable. This is why it's so important to start acknowledging how we are feeling daily. This exercise, which takes its name from the acronym RAIN (**R**ecognize, **A**ccept, **I**nvestigate and **N**on-identify), helps to teach us the core meaning of mindfulness.

It's a quick and easy tool that you can use to help manage and understand your emotions. It's important to be kind to yourself, especially when managing difficult emotions, and I find it comforting to place a hand on my heart during this exercise.

This triggers a reminder to pause before saying anything I don't mean in the heat of the moment to myself or others.

Here is an explanation of what each letter means in relation to mindful practice:

'R' for Recognize

- The first step is to recognize the emotion you are experiencing. This could be anything from feeling overwhelmed, resentful, to unsettled or frustrated.

- Gently and without judgement bring yourself into the present moment. Tune in to your mind and body, take a pause and ask yourself, 'What am I experiencing right now?'

- It might help to say the emotion, such as 'I am feeling overwhelmed'.

- By recognizing the emotion and giving it a name it allows us to be present and prevents us from being in denial about how we are truly feeling.

'A' for Accept, Acknowledge or Allow

This is about accepting the emotion and letting it be. When we experience difficult emotions a natural response is to want to push them away or try to ignore them, instead of simply acknowledging how we are feeling. We can very quickly get caught up in our thoughts and react on impulse, but by stepping back and allowing the emotion to be what it is, it may help to ease resistance and soften how we are feeling.

'I' for Investigate

Now that you have recognized and allowed the emotion you can start to gently investigate how it feels with questions such as:

- Why am I feeling this way?

- What do I need to support myself?

- Is there something that could have heightened the intensity of this emotion? – such as lack of sleep.

Asking ourselves these questions enables us to tune in to our emotions, helping us to become better equipped to recognize how we are feeling sooner. This creates healthier relationships with our emotions.

'N' for Non-identify

The idea behind 'non-identify' is to simply experience the emotion without being defined by it. It is remembering not to take our emotions personally, because they are not unique to us – they are shared by us all.

Remember not to label yourself with the emotion and instead be careful with the language that you use. Replace 'I am such a resentful person' with 'I am experiencing resentment'.

Underneath every thought there is a stillness we can reconnect to, allowing us a sense of freedom from unwanted feelings and emotions.

I have chosen a very simple example to show how I have found each letter of RAIN helpful. Lola and Kit have been pretty good eaters, but have both inevitably gone through fussy stages, which can make mealtimes challenging, especially as they copy each other's behaviour. I am sure we've all experienced spending a lot of time planning and preparing a meal for our children only for them to refuse to eat it. Nothing makes me feel more frustrated than when the bowls of food get pushed away and the words 'no' from Kit and 'I don't like it, Mummy' from Lola ring out around our kitchen!

I either have to make the choice for them to simply not eat (and go hungry) or prepare something else for them. Before you know it, you end up preparing individual meals for each member of the family – something I always promised myself I wouldn't do!

How can RAIN help us through frustration like this?

R – I recognized I was feeling frustrated.

> I brought myself into the moment,
> remembering that teatime is notoriously a
> time of day when we can all feel tetchy
> and tired and perhaps in need of peace
> and quiet.

A – I accepted the feeling of frustration and I was able to let it be.

> This step reminds me to put the emotion
> into perspective and try not to act on
> impulse. Having encouraged Lola and Kit
> to try a few mouthfuls, explaining that
> they need to eat so they can grow, I
> have learned to try my best to let go
> and move on!

I – This is when I investigate why my reaction
is feeling so intense.

Why am I feeling this way?
I spent time planning and preparing a
meal I hoped my children would enjoy.

What can I do to support myself?
Stay present, keep a sense of humour
and take a few deep breaths.

*Is there something that could have heightened
this emotion?*
A busy and demanding day with both the
children, in need of some time to myself.

N – It helps to remind myself that I share
this emotion with many others who have
experienced fussy eating and that frustration is shared by us all.

Using RAIN is a reminder to work through an
emotion before it escalates. It gives us time out
from the situation. And if all else fails at teatime,
once I've gone through RAIN, I reach for toast
and a banana. That never fails to win them over!

Letting go

'Some of us think holding on makes us
strong; but sometimes it is letting go.'
– Hermann Hesse

Having used control as a way of coping with anxiety
for many years, one of the biggest lessons, especially
during fertility treatment and motherhood, has been
learning to let go.

The more we hold on and think we are in control, the more out of control we can often be. I have
to remind myself daily that I can't control all aspects
of my life nor the children's. Every day something
different is thrown at us: a change of plan, one of
the children is poorly, the car has a flat tyre, there is
sudden extra admin that you hadn't planned for, a

family day trip that should be fun turns into a day of tears and tantrums, your child suddenly discovers they can climb the bigger climbing frame at the park, and so it goes on. There is always something unexpected and it is simply impossible to stay in control of everything.

The irony is that letting go of worries and control can help relieve anxiety, but I have found this takes a lot of practice and repetition. The more frustrated we feel and the more we try to cling on, the tougher life can feel. If we practise letting go, being flexible and going with the flow more, however hard this is for some of us, the weight of control and anxiety can start to lift and we can begin to give ourselves permission to feel freedom from the restrictions we have created because we think they are helping us cope.

All of us have worries and at times we can hold on to these anxious thoughts and give them too much space to grow in our minds. The internal chatter of 'what ifs' becomes our reality and we begin to lose focus on the situation, believing in the story we are creating and imagining.

For example, I know for me personally health worries can trigger anxiety. When I read or hear about people who are very unwell or if I'm informed of a sickness bug going around nursery, the fear becomes very real. Not knowing if it will happen and when or how it might happen and not having any control over the situation can bring on an episode of anxiety. We can find ourselves holding our breath in times of worry, so using a mindful breathing practice, such as the breathing cycle on page 26, can really help remind you to breathe, release fear and give you strength and courage to survive the intense moments of motherhood.

How to let go of unwanted emotions is a lesson we can teach our children. Opening up conversations and helping them understand that adults have worries too hopefully allows them to express their fears rather than hold on to them.

Here are some exercises to help us let go:

Bubbles

Lola and Kit, like many other children, love bubbles, so this is a simple way of explaining to a young child about letting go of worries.

Talk together about something that is troubling you, then imagine blowing that worry inside a bubble and, as the bubble disappears, let the worry go.

To watch something disappear is very visual. Encourage your children, if you can, not to pop the bubbles but to see them disappear or float away. This develops an understanding about patience and allows us to let something be without trying to change anything.

Watching bubbles is a calming way to focus our mind on the present and blowing bubbles encourages deep breathing, both of which promote a good mindful practice to share.

Worry box

Creating a worry box is a good way to open up a dialogue within the family about worries. By writing down your thoughts or encouraging your children to write theirs it not only helps them to understand their concerns more clearly, it is also very therapeutic. When they have finished writing down their worry they put the paper back in the box. Together, a few days later, you can go back to the box and read the worries and talk about whether it is still bothering them. If the worry has passed, you might choose to rip up the paper, letting go of it altogether, or if not you can put it back and check in on it another time. By sharing this exercise with your child it might encourage them to open up to you about what is troubling them.

Holding hands

Sit holding both hands with your child, squeezing your hands together and then releasing the tension in them. As you release you could say a sentence such as:

- I want to let go of feeling nervous.
- I want to calm down.
- I want to feel safe.
- All is calm.
- All is well.
- I am safe.

For mums

For mums letting go could just be taking a moment to think about what is making life complicated and asking if there is something you could let go of or remove to simplify your life and help bring back balance. Perhaps when adding something to your diary you remove something else so that life doesn't feel too crowded.

Letting go at the end of the day

Begin with some mindful breathing to settle yourself.

> Lying flat on your back in bed, imagine holding your worries and concerns inside the palm of your hands.

> Continue by opening up your hands and visualize the worries floating away, imagining physically letting them go, with the knowledge that after a good night's sleep and with a clearer mind in the morning you will be able to decide if these thoughts are still troubling you, if they need your attention or if you can let them go once and for all.

> This can help the weight of worry feel lighter at the end of the day and help to prepare the mind and body for a good night's sleep.

My mindful affirmation

At the start of the book I suggested setting a mindful affirmation for yourself. The one I use daily is 'Let go'.

> Take a moment right now to pause, feel your body and mind relax, take a slow breath in and think 'Let', and as you breathe out slowly think 'Go'.
>
> Repeat this as many times as you need.

Go to bed, Little one

One of the reasons I began exploring the benefits of mindfulness for children was to learn more about how mindful exercises could help Lola and Kit at bedtime, because I wanted to find something that would act like an emotional comfort blanket for them at night.

Having grown up with so much fear around going to bed, I wanted to have the tools to help Lola and Kit develop a healthy relationship with sleep, so they don't have to experience the anxieties that I still struggle with, but if they do, I want to educate myself about how to comfort and reassure them.

It is often when our head hits the pillow that our mind becomes active, wandering off in the silence with unwanted thoughts, which is why a mindful practice at bedtime is so powerful. Hopefully noticing habits from a young age about how our mind behaves will help change the pattern and give children knowledge about how to prepare for a good night's sleep.

Sleep plays an essential role in our children's development and research recommends a regular and consistent bedtime routine. Often our children have other ideas about a good night's sleep, which can leave us all feeling sleep-deprived. I have turned to the exercises below, such as the visualization story for support during night wakings, as I find not only do they soothe Lola and Kit, they also help to keep my mind quiet, so I can hopefully drift back off to sleep again too!

I hope some of the exercises below encourage bedtime to be a calm time for you and your children, and that it is a peaceful way to end the day together. I have also included an exercise for when we wake up in the morning to help start the day positively.

Remember not to worry if your child chooses not to engage in an exercise. Just try again another time.

Breathing

As an adult, practising breathing exercises has been the single most helpful way for me to ease anxiety, especially at bedtime. If we practise breathing at other times during the day, when we are less anxious, our mind can learn how to tap into a relaxed state more quickly when we need it most, such as during the quiet moments at night.

Start by settling your child down comfortably in bed and begin with some gentle breathing, such as Teddy breathing (see page 44) or Take five (see page 57).

Breathing gives us something to come back to when our mind begins to wander. The key is learning to notice our thoughts and then encouraging the mind back to the breath.

To help Lola understand this I explain what I might be thinking about, such as I need to pack your school bag for the morning. I then go on to ask her to imagine this thought like a cloud above her head and then ask her to watch it float away. Continue by going back to the breathing exercise you are sharing.

Although this might seem advanced to grasp when they are still young, as times goes on they begin to understand better and it will help develop their mindful practice.

Body scan

Please refer back to page 32 for detailed body scan (One-minute mindfulness).

Continuing on from settling down our breathing we can begin a short body scan with our child. This helps our children to calm down, relaxing the body and bringing a mindful awareness about how the body is feeling. This could be tired, achy or perhaps peaceful. It is an exercise you can practise together as a way to unwind.

- Begin by asking your child to wiggle their fingers and toes. This allows them to turn their attention to their body.

- Ask your child to imagine something soft, such as a feather or leaf, resting gently on their skin as you move through each part of the body, starting with the feet, followed by the legs, tummy, chest, arms, hands and face. As your child gets older you can be more detailed, such as knees and thighs, etc.

- As you move up the body ask your child if they can tense each part of the body and then let go. A way to practise this is by using a small squishy ball. Ask your child to squeeze it tightly and then let go. Continue by asking them to repeat the action without the ball. Although this might be tricky to understand for younger children, particularly with tensing areas such as the tummy and chest, as they grow older they will begin to gain an improved awareness about this sensation. With Lola being three I concentrate on her squeezing her toes, hands and face. It helps to demonstrate the action; scrunching up my face is Lola's favourite!

Visualization story – a peaceful place

The idea of this exercise is to remember a place or moment in time when you felt calm so that when you go back there it evokes the same feeling.

Once you have quietened down the mind with breathing and relaxed the body using a body scan you can begin to talk about your peaceful place.

This visualization story is one Lola and I created together called 'The Sleepy Meadow'. It feels like our very own bedtime story and is now part of our sleep routine.

We started by talking about somewhere that Lola felt happy and calm, which was at a local park that we often visit. We talked about who else might be there and the colours of the flowers, the grass, the different smells and other details, such as the waterfall and the bridge we walk over. You can keep adding to your story and explain that this is their happy and safe place where they can go to at any time; it is a place that is always waiting for them when they need it.

Our Sleepy Meadow script

'Lola and Mummy take the bus to our favourite place, the sleepy meadow. When we arrive it is very peaceful and the only people in our sleepy meadow are Mummy, Lola, Daddy and Kit. We walk down the stone steps and with each step we take a deep breath in and out and as we do we feel calmer and quieter. It is a warm day and the sun is sparkling through the branches of the trees. We take off our shoes and socks so we can feel the soft grass between our toes. We walk past the little waterfall and over the bridge before arriving at our favourite meadow. In the meadow we can smell the purple lavender and the green grass is filled with pretty daisies. We lie down together, holding hands peacefully in our meadow. Daddy and Kit go off to play but we decide to have a little rest. We put a light blanket over us and gently close our eyes. You are safe here in your sleepy meadow.'

For my own visualization story I remember a beach Harry and I visited on holiday a few years ago. I find this particularly relaxing at bedtime, especially when struggling to sleep. The sound of the waves, the sunset, the feeling of warm soft sand under my feet, the breeze from the trees, Harry beside me reading his book on the sunlounger. Remembering this place always gives me a feeling of ease, peace and contentment.

A comforter

When I was growing up I struggled going for sleepovers with friends as I always felt homesick. My mum used to give me one of her hankies and sprayed it with her perfume. This was so comforting and it was something I continued to use when I felt vulnerable or needed her support when we were apart.

Rainbow of friendship

This exercise gives children the chance to think of those they love before drifting off to sleep. It is a reminder to be grateful for what we have and to be thoughtful and kind to others.

We start by imagining each different colour of the rainbow connecting our heart to the heart of someone we love in the shape of a rainbow, linking us together.

We give each person their own colour and wish them love and happiness. We then send them something such as a wish or thank-you.

An example of Lola's rainbow wishes:

- **Red**: Daddy – thank you for taking me for a ride on my scooter.

- **Orange**: Granny – I hope the flowers in your garden made you smile today.

- **Yellow**: Kit – I hope you feel better in the morning so you don't have a runny nose any more.

- **Green**: Friends – I can't wait to share games with you at nursery tomorrow.

- **Blue**: Mummy – I hope you sleep well tonight.

- **Indigo**: Grandad – thank you for always reading me stories.

- **Violet**: Nursery teacher – thank you for painting with me today.

Sprinkles

Sprinkles is an exercise to help develop gratitude, awareness, friendship and love.

Rubbing your thumb and first two fingers together you can pretend to sprinkle magic over your friends and family. It is a chance to tell them something simple they have done that has helped you, made you happy or made you feel better.

For example:

- I sprinkle my mum for listening to me.

- I sprinkle my friend for sharing her snack with me.

- I sprinkle my granny for collecting me from school.

- I sprinkle my dad for playing games with me.

Lola and I use sprinkles in the night too if she wakes up. I tell her I am covering her in Mummy's magic sprinkles to keep her safe.

Wake up with the sun in your heart

In the morning as you wake up imagine a golden sun in your heart, feel the warm glow and picture the rays expanding through your body, giving you a sense of energy, strength, love and courage. You could also visualize the rays expanding to family or friends, giving them rays of energy for the day ahead.

At nighttime you can use the same technique, but visualizing the sunset and the beautiful soft colours. Allow the image of a sunset to help bring your body and mind into a state of relaxation.

- Start by finding a comfortable position – this can be standing, sitting or lying down.

- Take a few deep breaths, soften the body and gently close your eyes or lower your gaze.

- Place your left hand on your heart and your right hand on your abdomen.

- Notice the feeling of warmth from your hands on the body.

- You can slowly say the following phrases aloud or in your head: 'May you be happy, may you be healthy, may you be calm, may you be safe.'

- Take a moment to really absorb the words and repeat the phrases as many times as you would like.

- Finish with a few deep breaths.

You can replace the words 'happy', 'healthy', 'calm' and 'safe' with any words that feel right for you in that moment. 'Peaceful', 'patient', 'content' and 'relaxed' work really well too.

It feels special to practise the same exercise with Lola and to know I can also share it with Kit when he is older. When Lola is tucked up in bed at the end of the day we say these sentences out loud together. I was amazed to see a child as young as three responding so positively. It has been a helpful tool to settle Lola during the night, and at bedtime she will often start these sentences without me prompting her, so I can see Lola finds it comforting too. It's very calming for us both to share these words before turning out the lights.

You can adapt the exercise to practise with your child as follows:

- Start by finding a comfortable position, somewhere your child can feel calm and relaxed. I practise this exercise with Lola when she is settling down to go to sleep, so usually lying down.

- Take a few deep breaths together. You can encourage this by saying, 'Breathe in and breathe out.'

- Place one hand on your child's heart and ask them to place one hand on your heart. At this point I talk to Lola about how our hearts are connected and that she is safe.

- Then you can slowly say the phrases together: 'May you be happy, may you be healthy, may you be calm, may you be safe.'

Once again, you can replace the words here with whatever feels appropriate for you and your child. I often use 'May you sleep well'. (Worth a try for a good night's sleep!)

Having spent my childhood with anxieties about going to sleep, mainly based around the fear of being alone, I think this type of exercise would have been really beneficial. This is why I focus attention on feeling safe when I practise this with Lola and Kit in the hope that it gives them reassurance to feel confident and calm at night when they go to sleep.

I hope that in the years to come Lola and Kit will share this exercise together and continue to use it by themselves. I like the idea that even when we are apart, if we are each continuing to do this, we will think of one another and it will connect us as a family, giving reassurance and comfort to us all.

Self-care

Let's talk about self-care

♡

'Self-care is not self-indulgent;
self-care is self-respect.'

Self-care is anything that improves physical, emotional and mental well-being. Regular self-care practice has been shown to lower stress levels, improve health and is one of the most positive choices you can make for yourself.

Self-care is not selfish. It is not a luxury. It is essential. We can spend so much of our time punishing ourselves rather than nourishing ourselves. Our lives become so busy and full that we forget to create time for the most important person – you!

For many mums time for well-being is the last

thing on our list and yet we should really be prioritizing ourselves rather than being an afterthought at the end of a day. Being a mum at times is relentless, constantly doing things for others with a mental overload that never seems to end. Self-care isn't just one thing, like a cup of tea in peace (however wonderful that feels!); it's looking at our holistic approach to well-being. As a mum, remembering who you are and what is important to you is something that shouldn't be neglected or pushed to one side. It is important to acknowledge just how capable we are and to let go of thinking we are somehow failing or not doing a good enough job. The relentlessness of motherhood and our ability to just cope and get on with it, accepting tiredness and busyness, becomes our normal. We are constantly putting others first, often forgetting to pay attention to our own needs before we become burnt out, exhausted and no good to anyone, especially ourselves.

We all have an idea about what self-care might look like for us but it's important to remember that this can be different for everyone. Whatever self-care looks like to you, we should all accept it as part of a lifestyle choice without judgement towards yourself or others. It is important to allow yourself this time without any guilt attached to it.

I have learned that little pockets of self-care throughout the day go a long way. I enjoy taking exercise and try to walk when I can rather than take the car for errands so I can be outside. Nutritious food, listening to music, taking time to rest and spending time with friends all help to improve my overall mood and give me the energy I need to feel recharged and ready to step back into the toughest and most rewarding job of all, being a mum.

If we surround ourselves with all that is good in our lives, spending time creating an environment where we feel calm, safe and relaxed with the people who make us feel loved and happy, this is nourishment and this is self-care.

To start, here are ten self-care thoughts:

1. Remember self-care is different for everyone. Take time to think about what it is you need to support and nourish you.

2. Learn to prioritize yourself without any guilt. We all need a chance to recharge and to have time for ourselves.

3. Set your boundaries and don't be afraid to say no.

4. It feels good to give someone you care about time for themselves too. For example, take it in turns with a friend to have each other's children for an afternoon so you can both have some time for yourself.

5. Listen to your inner wisdom. If it's time to take a break or things are getting on top of you, don't be afraid to ask for help.

6. Make it part of your routine to schedule time in your diary for yourself.

7. Give yourself a digital detox and switch off for a while.

8. Take time to slow down and learn what the warning signs are when you start to feel overwhelmed. It's OK to stop and simply do nothing sometimes. See Nothing time on page 71.

9. Practising mindfulness, going to a yoga class or taking a walk are all positive ways to relax and check back in with ourselves.

10. Speak kindly to yourself. Remember: nourish don't punish!

Looking after your health and well-being doesn't need to be expensive, and even finding pockets of time during the day for self-care is beneficial. The following exercises are simple yet effective, and they also include ways to help reconnect you with the things you love.

Tired eyes

This is a simple and quick exercise that you can use any time of day. It is also useful to use after long periods of screen time. We all have thirty seconds to spare somewhere in our day to enjoy this little treat.

- Rub your hands together quickly until they feel warm.

- Cup your hands over your eyes and take in the stillness, darkness and warmth from your hands.

- Allow the tension around your eyes to drift away and use the moment to relax and take a few mindful breaths.

Face relaxation

This is an exercise to add in to the start and end of each day. It's using the moments we already have to give ourselves something back. It only takes seconds but it feels like a warm hug!

As you moisturize your face massage the cream into the skin with your hands. Use this as a chance to release tension in the face, paying attention to the areas where we tend to hold more tension, such as the jaw, cheeks, temples and between the eyes.

You can also apply this method when moisturizing your neck and shoulders. Take the opportunity to give yourself a gentle massage, letting the tension of the day ease and use this as a reminder to relax your shoulders.

Hand on your heart

The simplicity of this exercise is what is so beautiful about it.

Often when we are touched by something that moves us emotionally a natural response is to want to touch our heart with our hands. This soothing and comforting action releases the happy hormone oxytocin, so soak this up as much as you can.

I find myself reaching for this first thing in the morning before I begin my day, during challenging times or during those difficult moments with the little ones when you hear the word 'no' and 'why' a few too many times! It reminds us to be patient, to trust and be kind with ourselves. This simple action is always available to you as a gentle reminder to take care of yourself.

- As you place your hand on your heart you can choose to add a sentence to help calm or relax you. I often say the words 'All is calm, all is well, I am safe' or 'Everything is OK' or 'This too shall pass'.

- Placing your other hand on top, feel your heart beating and the warmth from your hands.

- Closing your eyes or lowering your gaze, take some cleansing breaths in through the nose and out through the mouth.

- Allow yourself to just be.

Practising this action regularly helps teach us the sensation of feeling calm and gives us a moment to give back to ourselves.

Gift for the day

Give yourself a gift each day, a promise to yourself of something nurturing just for you. This could be some flowers, a bubble bath, an episode of your favourite TV programme, a walk on your own, your favourite chocolate, a yoga class. This is a gentle act of kindness and self-care.

Going back to something you love

This was something I discovered during fertility treatment. A realization that I had forgotten to take care of the interests and hobbies that gave me confidence and happiness but most importantly reminded me who I was. Just as it had felt during fertility treatment, in the early days of motherhood it can be very easy to lose track of who you are; suddenly your identity changes, and that left me feeling quite alone and lost. The going back to something I loved for me was music, so I decided to join an amateur orchestra so I could play my violin once a week. I had lost all confidence to play professionally, but being surrounded by others who were simply enjoying their music-making was enough for me.

Reconnecting with something you love is incredibly powerful. It not only helps to remind us who we are, it also shows us that being a mum doesn't mean we have to lose our identity. We still deserve time to enjoy our interests and hobbies, and these shouldn't be forgotten in the chaos of motherhood.

I have started to look for ways to bring my passion for music into my family's life and use it as an opportunity to share something I love with Lola and Kit. I now play my violin to the children, usually at around 5.30 p.m., when everyone is exhausted and grizzly. I find music a wonderful way to turn a toddler's whinge into a smile, and it calms everyone down, including me!

Sharing my love of music helps me stay connected with it. I play music in the house and talk about anything music-related with the children as I feel it's important that they understand how much music means to me. I might sing the words to a book at story time and sing my way through pretty much everything! I make up songs during mealtimes about the wonders of vegetables, during bath time about soapy water in their hair and at bedtime to gently soothe them to sleep. Music is magical and I'm so grateful to be able to share my love for it with my children every day. See the music exercises in Sharing mindful moments with your family on page 213.

Whatever your love is, the most important thing is to reconnect with it. So perhaps ask yourself what joy you have lost touch with and whether there is something that could reconnect you with it?

'Find what makes your heart sing and
create your own music.' – Mac Anderson

Looking after yourself in the early days of motherhood

♡

'Strength grows in the moments
when you think you can't get on but you
keep going anyway.'

Having gone through the heartache of trying to conceive, undergoing IVF treatment and suffering a devastating miscarriage, I hadn't given myself the chance to really think about what life would be like when our baby was born. I spent my pregnancies feeling fearful that things wouldn't be OK. I was afraid to imagine becoming a mum, but in those brief moments when I dared to think about it I naively assumed that as soon as I held my baby all my worries would disappear.

The pure love and total relief I felt when holding Lola in my arms for the first time was magical. Looking back, I now realize that having focused so much on a healthy pregnancy I failed to prepare myself emotionally for the reality of motherhood and the huge responsibility and change that comes with it. Becoming a mum was a shock. During the first night after Lola was born I remember lying in bed staring at her with the sudden realization of just how fragile we both were. It felt like it was just the two of us in the world, but a world that was brand new in every way.

From the day Lola arrived into my life I felt vulnerable. In my arms was a baby I knew I loved completely and yet I didn't know her at all. I didn't know how she liked to be held, I was confused about when and how to feed her, I didn't know how to breastfeed, I didn't know how to swaddle her or if she even liked being swaddled. I didn't know how to wash or dress her without her crying and I had never changed a nappy. I remember thinking that I was no good at this already, and it quickly became all about survival and simply getting to the end of the day. A feeling of failure set in so early on and I was ashamed to admit to family and friends that I needed help. I thought I should be able to cope, just as it seemed every other mum around me was doing. The only way I could describe it was like being a duck that on the surface looked like it was gliding along effortlessly, but underneath its feet were paddling furiously trying to keep up.

Along with all these feelings I was recovering physically from giving birth while emotionally sitting in a hormonal fog, feeling every emotion from frustration to love. My breasts were engorged and incredibly sore from breastfeeding while leaking milk all over the place, mainly through my tops when friends and family came to visit. I was glued to my breastfeeding app to help remind me which side I had fed from last and obsessing about how long Lola was feeding for. I was constantly hungry and thirsty and the night sweats went on and on (no one tells you about those). I couldn't understand how something so small could need so much and stop you being able to manage even the basics of having a shower in the morning or eating a meal before it went cold. I was scared about how it was possible to leave the house with a newborn (surely it was safer to stay at home than risk the possibility

of a screaming baby in public!) and when I did ven-
ture out I would often end up walking home joining
in with Lola's tears. During the quiet moments I
felt alone – even though I had the amazing strength
and support from Harry.

If there was any advice I could go back and tell
myself, it would have been to have had more belief
in my own instinct and to have had the courage to
only take on board the advice and opinions that felt
right for me and not someone else. To have felt able
to admit when I was struggling and to have asked
and accepted help from family and friends. To have
talked about finding it hard without feeling ashamed
or guilty for experiencing anything other than joy
and realizing it was OK to stay at home until I felt
ready to leave the house. I feel I could have made
more preparations for myself to manage such a
life-changing moment and spent time thinking
about what I might need to put in place to support
me. Above all, a mother's love is unique and powerful, so I should have listened to and trusted my
heart more, something I'm still learning to do.

According to research, a feeling of failure is shared
by two thirds of British parents in the first year of
parenting, which is why having open and honest
conversations about the reality of parenthood is so

important. As the saying goes, 'It takes a village to raise a child'; however, unlike in previous generations, we are living at such a different pace, with the added pressures of things like social media and all the while wrestling expectations to raise a family, run a home and work all at once. We simply don't have the same immediate support. We prepare for other big life events, such as preparing to move house or for a job interview, so I think there is plenty we can proactively do to prepare ourselves for motherhood. We can put our safety blankets in place, and create our own village in preparation for one of the biggest and most overwhelming changes you will ever experience in your life.

*Help and support**

Ask for help. If you find this hard, in advance of your due date take time to think about who your support network is and who you can call on if you need to. It is natural to want to do everything yourself, but this can leave you feeling exhausted, especially while

* For more help and support visit the charity Tommy's website at: www.tommys.org/pregnancy-information/health-professionals/ free-pregnancy-resources/pregnancy-and-post-birth-wellbeing-plan

physically recovering and trying to manage the rollercoaster of emotions that comes with the surge of hormones. Letting go of control and accepting support is the first step, and it might be worth talking with your partner about your shared needs and what you feel you might need assistance with. That could be more help around the house, a food shop, preparing a meal, looking after the baby while you have a nap, finding local support groups – all of these are positive steps.

It might also be worth thinking about a family member or friend that you can ask to check in with you, perhaps once a week, for a chat to talk about how you are getting on.

Relationships

I think a good place to start is to discuss with your partner not only how you can help each other during the day but also about how to manage the disturbed nights. A few weeks in, Harry and I decided that I would do the night feeds but he would get up with Lola in the morning so I could catch up on sleep, which worked for us both. As we got into the swing of things Harry would always make sure at night that he would leave a glass of water and a snack bar on my bedside table, ready for when I suddenly felt ravenously hungry and thirsty while up feeding Lola. In the early days I think at times Harry felt quite helpless as so much demand was naturally on me. I realized a few weeks in that small gestures like running a bath, making a cup of tea or cooking dinner meant the world to me, and it was important to communicate that with him.

I think it's also important to talk about who is going to visit and when. Harry wanted the world and his wife to come and visit us whereas I would have been quite happy to have waited a good few weeks! It's important to think about this in advance, finding a compromise and setting the boundaries that you both feel comfortable with.

Sleep and screens

Prioritize your sleep! As we all know sleep deprivation can have a huge impact on our overall well-being. I remember feeling like I wanted to spend time in the evening with Harry as I missed our time together, just the two of us. The reality, though, was that dinner became a juggling act as we tried to soothe a restless baby. Sometimes when I did go to bed early I would lie there asking myself if I did go to sleep would I feel worse having to wake up in only an hour. I would often be waiting for Lola to wake and if she didn't, I would then feel frustrated that I hadn't gone to sleep. Prioritizing an early night is vital and it still is now that my children are toddlers!

Listening to podcasts or audiobooks can be great company and a good alternative to looking at your phone screen, which as we know can make it harder to fall back to sleep. I found the Headspace app helpful when trying to get back to sleep after a night feed too.

Well-being

Take care of your own well-being and ask yourself what you need to allow you to feel better. It could be organizing a gentle walk with a friend, asking your partner to plan healthy meal options or finding the time to rest and relax.

Drinking plenty of water and nourishing yourself with good food can help with exhaustion and will also aid your body in recovery. Tiredness can make you crave sugar, so perhaps have some healthier alternatives stocked up. Set your boundaries and never stop looking after yourself. Don't be afraid to put yourself first.

Mindfulness

Bringing your mind back to the present moment is so powerful. Using the breathing exercises in this book will help you to find your inner calm.

It's easy to wish away each stage, willing your baby to reach the next milestone, so taking a mindful pause will help to soak up the magical moment you are sharing with your baby.

Hearing your baby cry can make you instinctively feel stressed, and your natural response is to want to soothe them. Kit had terrible silent reflux as a baby and there were days when the relentless noise of his cry became so unbearable I would feel myself becoming tense, frustrated and upset that I couldn't seem to do anything to comfort him. During these moments it helped to consciously stop for a mindful breath and to physically release the tension in my body. I found it helpful to drop my shoulders, and relax the tension around my eyes and jaw.

There are many exercises in this book that you can practise to support you through these challenging moments, such as Calm begins with me (see page 53) and One-minute mindfulness (see page 29). Perspective in motherhood (see page 197) and WAIT (see page 68) might also be useful.

Affirmations

With the help of notes you can place affirmations around your home as a mindful reminder to support and reassure you. While reading the affirmation pause for a mindful breath.

- I will take care of myself.

- It's OK to ask for help.

- When there is chaos around me I am the calm.

- I will do all I can.

- Motherhood is challenging for everyone.

- Whatever I do today will be enough.

- This too shall pass.

- I must take care of myself so I can take care of those I love.

- Taking time for me is not only OK, it is essential.

Sleep

♡

Sleep is as important to us as breathing, eating and drinking. It is a vital ingredient in maintaining good mental and physical health and yet can often be neglected when considering our overall well-being. Lack of sleep can impact our mood and make us feel irritable. It affects our motivation and ability to make decisions, and can leave us reaching for unhealthy foods for that quick fix.

We spend a third of our lives asleep and yet I often put sleep at the bottom of my list of priorities, instead thinking of all the jobs I could be getting done once the children are in bed and trying to tick everything off my never-ending to-do list rather than heading to bed at a sensible time. Reminding ourselves that some jobs can wait and that our time doesn't always need to be filled isn't easy as a busy mum. It can feel like there is a constant need to catch up on sleep; Harry and I often joke about the amount of time we spend telling each other how tired we are, and I've lost count of the messages sent between friends saying it would be lovely to wake up one morning and not feel exhausted! Even knowing the importance of an early night and with my inner voice telling me 'You're tired, go to bed,' I still crave and value my alone time in the evening when the house is peaceful.

Since becoming a mum I've realized how tough it can be when you feel tired to remain calm and rational. Our patience can be seriously tested, especially when our tank is running on empty. I remember when Lola was born and being asked many times 'Is she a good sleeper?' I was very fortunate that Lola did sleep well, but I would often reply saying that she did but that my sleep was terrible! I was always conscious that I was needed, and especially when my children were tiny babies I was fearful that they were not OK. I couldn't rest because I wanted to keep an eye on them.

I struggle to completely switch off at bedtime and fall into a deep sleep. I have, however, decided that it is crucial that I set aside a couple of nights a week to go to bed early, so this is now part of my to-do list.

Here are some suggestions for how to prepare your mind and body for a relaxing night's sleep:

- Warm bath

  Running a warm foamy bath raises your body temperature, then as your body begins to cool down afterwards this helps you feel sleepy.

- Nighttime cuppa

  It's good to avoid caffeine and alcohol as these are stimulants that can interfere with falling asleep, but enjoying a night-time herbal tea can aid restful sleep.

- A sanctuary

  Make your bedroom a sanctuary that you feel comfortable in. Fill your room with things you love, such as photographs of loved ones and artwork that helps you feel peaceful. Why not indulge in some luxury bedding?

- Happy thoughts

  Try keeping a notepad by your bed to
  write down any concerns or thoughts
  that are on your mind. It might be a
  helpful way to let go of the worries,
  knowing you can go back to your notes
  the next day. Perhaps finish your writing
  with something you felt grateful for that
  day and try to consciously make your last
  thoughts of the day happy ones.

- Calm

  Scents such as lavender or geranium can
  help relax the mind and body. A few
  drops of essentials oils on your pillow
  can make you feel calmer. It might also
  be comforting to use a bath oil and body
  cream with a scent you find relaxing.

- Visualization

  Imagine yourself lying on a tropical beach
  with the warm sun in the sky, soft sand
  beneath you, listening to the gentle sound
  of the sea and waves lapping on the shore.
  Take a moment to tune in with your

senses, visualizing the colours of the beach, the sound of the sea and the way the sand feels between your fingertips.

Allow your body to feel heavy as you soak up the paradise you have created around you. Allow this peaceful place to help you drift off into a restful sleep.

Other activities that can help you unwind your busy mind include doing a body scan (see page 32), a mindful breathing cycle (see page 25), considering screen boundaries (see page 182) and letting go at the end of the day (see page 88).

Water

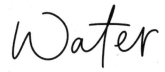

It is recommended that we drink six to eight glasses of water per day. I'm always conscious about Lola and Kit drinking enough water, but often need to remind myself to do the same, so in the morning when filling up the children's water bottles I fill up a large bottle for myself.

There are many benefits to drinking water that help our health and state of mind. Here are some reasons to stay hydrated:

- It helps us to feel refreshed, focused and alert.

- Dehydration can cause a negative impact on our mood and also affect our attention span and memory.

- Water helps aid good digestion.
- Going without water for too long can cause headaches.
- Sometimes when we feel tired or hungry it could be that we are actually dehydrated. Filling ourselves back up with water could help zap the sleepiness or hunger.

Drinking lemon water

I introduced warm water with lemon juice into my daily routine when it was suggested that it is good for the nervous system as lemon contains potassium. It is thought that anxiety and depression are often a result of low levels of potassium, so given that I suffer from anxiety I'm always willing to try anything that might help. I have also learned that drinking caffeine first thing can trigger adrenaline, which can contribute to anxiety, so I have found that lemon water is a better way for me to start the day.

It is thought that the biggest benefit may not be

from the lemon but actually the temperature of the water. Drinking any water, especially warm water, can help flush the digestive system, rehydrate the body and increase energy levels. Moreover, lemon contains vitamin C, an essential nutrient to maintain good health, so here are some of the benefits to starting your day with lemon and warm water:

- Cleanses and aids digestion

  Cleanses and flushes the digestive system.

- Immune system

  The vitamin C in lemon gives our immune system a boost – very important for us busy mums trying to avoid the children's viruses!

- Good for your mood

  Typically we haven't consumed any water for at least eight hours while sleeping, so starting the day with water is a great way to get the mind and body going. The scent of lemon is mood-enhancing and energizing and, as explained above, the potassium in lemon can help support the nervous system.

- Happier skin

  In helping improve digestion and because lemon contains vitamin C, it can also contribute to healthier skin.

After drinking warm water and lemon, swish some plain water in your mouth for about thirty seconds to make sure the citric acid from the lemon juice doesn't remain on the teeth.

Chakras

♡

Everyone has seven chakras, which are located in the midline of our body, and they are all connected to an energy centre. Each chakra has an individual colour and represents something different.

If you have attended a yoga or meditation class, it is likely that you have come across the word before. Personally it was during fertility treatment that I discovered a chakra meditation, which I found deeply relaxing and powerful. The sacral chakra is responsible for our sexual and creative energy and is located below the abdomen. I visualized the sun rising up from the sea. For me this symbolized new beginnings and hope, both of which comforted me during our difficulties to conceive.

I also have a weakness in my throat and have

suffered with tonsillitis regularly and on a few occasions lost my voice, so I have found the information below about the throat chakra helpful.

It is likely that some information about each individual chakra will resonate with you more than another.

Root chakra

Position: base of spine.
Colour: red.
Represents: grounding and trust.
Affirmation: 'I am.'

About:
The root chakra forms our foundation and represents the element earth. It helps to stabilize and support us and when functioning correctly we feel safe, grounded and able to let go of fear.

When it is blocked symptoms include:
PHYSICALLY: anxiety, issues connected to immune system, problems with legs, knees and feet.

EMOTIONALLY: sense of emptiness, disconnected, impatience, feeling alone.

Ways to help unblock the root chakra:

YOGA: mountain pose or any pose that helps you find stability.

MEDITATION: focus on feeling supported and safe; imagine yourself as strong as a tree with roots grounding you into the earth.

ELEMENT: earth, being around nature and enjoying walks.

BENEFICIAL FOODS: red foods, such as strawberries, red apples and tomatoes. Root vegetables, such as carrots, parsnips, beetroot. Proteins, such as eggs and nuts are very nourishing for the root chakra.

BALANCING THE ROOT CHAKRA: spend as much time as you can with people who help you feel supported. Enjoy the outdoors and being around nature. Being barefoot so you can connect with the ground.

A MINDFUL PRACTICE FOR THE ROOT CHAKRA: How to feel more grounded when your head is in the clouds (see page 49).

Sacral chakra

Position: lower abdomen.

Colour: orange.

Represents: sexuality and creativity.

Affirmation: 'I feel.'

About:

The sacral chakra is responsible for our sexual and creative energy and represents the element water. When functioning correctly you will feel able to express yourself emotionally and be able to connect with others.

When it is blocked symptoms include:

PHYSICALLY: lower back pains, fertility issues, complications with hips or thighs, bladder and kidney infections.

EMOTIONALLY: fear of change, emotional instability, uninspired creatively, lack of self-confidence.

Ways to help unblock the sacral chakra:

YOGA: triangle pose or any pose that opens your hips.

146

MEDITATION: imagine a beautiful orange sunrise on the water and focus on accepting change and new beginnings.

ELEMENT: water, being near water or enjoying a bath, going swimming.

BENEFICIAL FOODS: drink plenty of fluids and orange foods, including carrot, sweet potato and oranges.

BALANCING THE SACRAL CHAKRA: let go of difficult relationships and focus on hobbies that make you feel creative and happy.

A MINDFUL PRACTICE FOR THE SACRAL CHAKRA: RAIN (see page 77).

Solar plexus chakra

Position: upper abdomen.

Colour: yellow.

Represents: confidence and wisdom.

Affirmation: 'I can.'

About:

The solar plexus is our energy centre and represents the element fire. This chakra physically manages the nervous system and emotionally it provides us with self-esteem, self-discipline and strength. When functioning correctly it allows us to make decisions and trust our gut instinct.

When it is blocked symptoms include:

PHYSICALLY: gut health, digestive issues, diabetes.

EMOTIONALLY: procrastination, lack of confidence, sense of powerlessness.

Ways to help unblock the solar plexus chakra:

YOGA: any poses that strengthen the core such as the plank position.

MEDITATION: visualize a warm yellow light radiating around your body giving you strength and energy.

ELEMENT: fire – this element represents light, heat and energy. Enjoy soaking up the sunshine.

BENEFICIAL FOODS: eat foods that release energy slowly, such as oats and whole grains. Spices such as ginger, cinnamon and turmeric. Yellow foods, including banana, pineapple and lemon.

BALANCING THE SOLAR PLEXUS CHAKRA: hot yoga class, a walk in the sunshine or relaxing in a sauna. Anything with heat is your friend.

A MINDFUL PRACTICE FOR THE SOLAR PLEXUS CHAKRA: Wake up with the sun in your heart (see page 101).

Heart chakra

Position: heart centre.
Colour: green.
Represents: love and healing.
Affirmation: 'I love.'

About:
The heart chakra radiates love, joy and compassion and represents the element air. It is the chakra that connects the lower chakras to the upper chakras and when functioning correctly it allows us to love and accept ourselves so we are able to truly love others.

When it is blocked symptoms include:
PHYSICALLY: poor circulation, heart conditions, high/low blood pressure.
EMOTIONALLY: sadness, anger or greed.

Ways to help unblock the heart chakra:
YOGA: back bends like cobra or any pose that opens the heart.

MEDITATION: imagine yourself outside and feel the green grass between your toes. Concentrate on your breathing.

ELEMENT: air, being in the outdoors and around greenery.

BENEFICIAL FOODS: foods full of green goodness, including spinach, broccoli, avocado, kiwi, green apples and grapes. Green herbs, such as mint, coriander, basil and tarragon. Green superfoods, including green tea, matcha and spirulina.

BALANCING THE HEART CHAKRA: being outside and immersing yourself in nature, breathing in fresh air. When practising mindfulness focus on breathing exercises.

A MINDFUL PRACTICE FOR THE HEART CHAKRA: May you be (see page 103).

Throat chakra

Position: throat.
Colour: blue.
Represents: self-expression and communication.
Affirmation: 'I speak.'

About:

The throat chakra is related to self-expression and represents sound. It is the first of the higher chakras and when functioning correctly allows us to speak truthfully and honestly. It is also associated with listening and hearing and is an essential role for positive communication.

When it is blocked symptoms include:

PHYSICALLY: sore throat, cough, grinding teeth and stiff neck.

EMOTIONALLY: lack of creative expression, indecisiveness, difficulty in accepting criticism.

Ways to help unblock the throat chakra:

YOGA: fish pose or any pose that opens and strengthens the throat.

MEDITATION: visualize a soft blue scarf resting gently on the throat and while breathing out imagine a soft blue ribbon flowing out with the breath, giving you confidence to communicate truthfully.

ELEMENT: sound, listen to the calming sound of a peaceful ocean.

BENEFICIAL FOODS: liquids can help heal and soothe the throat chakra, such as soup, herbal tea, smoothies and juices. There aren't too many blue foods, but you could blend blueberries or blackberries into a smoothie.

BALANCING THE THROAT CHAKRA: singing . . . I use this as a good excuse to sing with the children or loudly in the car! Drink plenty of water. Take the time each day to speak truthfully and to really listen to others.

A MINDFUL PRACTICE FOR THE THROAT CHAKRA: Truly lisening (see page 205).

Third-eye chakra

Position: forehead, between the eyebrows.
Colour: indigo.
Represents: focusing and seeing the big picture.
Affirmation: 'I see.'

About:

The third eye is our intuition and represents light. When functioning correctly we are able to focus on seeing everything clearly and have a better imagination. It is believed that people with a balanced third-eye chakra have psychic abilities.

When it is blocked symptoms include:

PHYSICALLY: problems with your vision, hormonal imbalance, insomnia, dizziness.

EMOTIONALLY: out of touch with reality, ignore your intuition, obsessive, lost in thoughts, find it hard to be open-minded.

Ways to help unblock the third-eye chakra:

YOGA: eagle pose or any pose that encourages focus and concentration.

MEDITATION: gently close your eyes and focus your attention on a warm light in the centre of your eyebrows. Relax the muscles around your eyes and imagine the light softening into an indigo glow expanding out of the room, widening your perspective and opening your mind to see the bigger picture in a difficult situation you might be experiencing.

ELEMENT: light, enjoy the relaxation from candle-light, or practise meditation under sunlight or moonlight.

BENEFICIAL FOODS: dark chocolate has many health benefits, including increasing serotonin levels (the happy hormone). It also contains magnesium, which helps to relax and relieve stress. Other foods include purple foods, such as aubergine, grapes and purple kale. Omega-3-rich foods, such as salmon, nuts and chia seeds, boost brain power and therefore also support the third-eye chakra.

BALANCING THE THIRD-EYE CHAKRA: It is important to get enough sleep to rest the third eye and also to try to avoid too much screen time, especially before bed. Listen to your intuition and be imaginative.

A MINDFUL PRACTICE FOR THE THIRD-EYE CHAKRA: Tired eyes (see page 115).

Crown chakra

Position: top of head.
Colour: purple or white.
Represents: connection and spirituality.
Affirmation: 'I understand.'

About:

The crown chakra is our most spiritual chakra and represents connection with yourself and others. When functioning correctly you radiate gratitude and joy, and have an ability to let go of your ego.

When it is blocked symptoms include:

PHYSICALLY: headaches, depression, exhaustion, disorders of nervous system.

EMOTIONALLY: living in your thoughts, feeling disconnected from your body, selfish behaviour, lack of purpose.

Ways to help unblock the crown chakra:

YOGA: while practising yoga set an intention, such as 'I am connected' or 'I am fully present'.

MEDITATION: this is the chakra that requires us to practise meditation regularly so we can take some time for peace and quiet in our busy lives.

ELEMENT: thought.

BENEFICIAL FOODS: it is considered that there isn't a specific food type for the crown chakra. This could be because it is the most spiritual and more about mental rather than physical nourishment.

BALANCING THE CROWN CHAKRA: practising mindfulness in our day-to-day lives and using calming essential oils, such as lavender.

A MINDFUL PRACTICE FOR THE CROWN CHAKRA: Gratitude (see page 247).

A simple chakra meditation

To start, visualize a red light as you sit in a chair with your feet in front of you on the ground and breathe out trust.

- As you continue, touch each point with your first two fingers and take mindful breaths in and out.

- Visualize an orange light in the lower abdomen – breathe out acceptance.

- Visualize a yellow light in the upper abdomen – breathe out confidence.

- Visualize a green light in the centre of your heart – breathe out love and compassion.

- Visualize a blue light in the centre of your throat – breathe out words of kindness, truth and courage.

- Visualize an indigo light in your third eye – breathe out and focus on perspective.

- Visualize a purple light at the top of your head – breathe out and feel present.

- Visualize a red light in the base of your spine and allow yourself to feel peaceful and grounded as you come to the end of your meditation practice.

Going outside

The weather and emotions

♡♡

'You can't have a rainbow
without a little rain.'

The weather is something we start to observe and
talk about with children from a young age. Simply
talking about the weather is a very mindful way to
introduce an understanding about emotions.

We can use the weather to describe how we are
feeling and we can use it to teach children that we all
experience different emotions. We can explain that,
just like the weather, the way we are feeling comes
and goes, constantly changing, nothing staying the
same.

Changes to the weather can happen suddenly or

subtly, just like our mood. How we feel can be triggered by an immediate situation or something building up over time.

For example, someone jumping the queue to push in front of you could cause sudden irritation, whereas a friend who isn't being very thoughtful could become upsetting over time.

In a moment of sudden change to our mood we might choose to use an exercise such as Calm begins with me (see page 53) or WAIT (see page 68), which allow us the opportunity to pause and consider our reaction when challenged by an emotion.

When considering subtle changes it helps to have an awareness about how we feel before it becomes too upsetting or overwhelming. Using mindful techniques, such as THINK (see page 69) and RAIN (see page 77), helps us pay attention to our emotions and gives us the confidence to communicate and understand our feelings, while asking ourselves what we need to support us.

There are several exercises involving emotions that you can try with your children.

Learning about different emotions

With your child think of words to describe the different emotions and the type of weather that could correspond with them to help explain that feeling. Some suggestions include:

- Sunshine – happy/joy
- Rain – sad/upset
- Cloudy – worried
- Windy – frustration
- Foggy – lonely/lost
- Storm – angry/scared
- Rainbow – peaceful/calm
- Snow – excitement/wonder

Once you have settled on the descriptions discuss with your children when they might have experienced these emotions. For example, snow – excited for Christmas; foggy – starting a new school, new environment and making new friends; sunshine – on holiday and enjoying ice cream on the beach.

It is important for children to also hear about the times we have experienced different emotions. Here are some examples I have shared with Lola: rainbow – reading my book in peace with a cup of tea; windy – when Daddy forgot his house keys (again!); rain – when we had to say goodbye to our cat, Murphy.

If you continue to investigate these experiences further, ask your child how being happy makes their body feel. Do they have butterflies in their stomach or a smile or giggle that they can't take off their face?

You can adopt the same approach when they are feeling upset or angry. Does their stomach feel tight or is it difficult to smile?

Helping our children discover how the body responds to feelings, just as much as the mind does, allows them to make a link between the two. This is a very helpful way to bring a mindful awareness about the mind and body being connected.

A short guided meditation

- Sit comfortably and gently close your eyes.

- Let your body feel soft like a fluffy cloud.

- Take a deep breath in and imagine a round golden sunshine filling up your belly.

- As you breathe out imagine the beautiful colours of the rainbow flowing out of your mouth.

- How do you feel today? Are you happy like the sunshine?

- Can you see the sunshine? Can you feel the warmth from the sunshine? Just like feeling happy comes and goes, so do sunny days.

- Maybe you feel a bit worried like a cloud?

- Can you see a blanket of clouds in the sky? Can you feel the cool air? Just like feeling worried comes and goes, so does a cloudy day.

- Do you feel like the rain is heavy and are you feeling sad?

- Can you hear the rain falling? Can you see the droplets of rain on your window?

Just like feeling sad comes and goes, so does a rainy day.

• Are you calm and peaceful like a rainbow?

• Can you see the shape of a rainbow?
  Can you imagine all the different colours?
  Just like feeling calm comes and goes,
  so does a rainbow.

• Now think about the weather and how it changes every day. We might not feel how we want to sometimes, but our emotions come and go like the weather. How we feel will pass because nothing stays the same. We accept the rainy days as well as the sunny days. They are all part of our wonderful life.

• Now take a deep breath in and imagine a round golden sunshine filling up your belly.

• As you breathe out imagine the beautiful colours of the rainbow flowing out of your mouth.

• Wiggle your fingers and toes and slowly open your eyes.

Let's talk emotion

With your child sit and listen to each other and share three emotions you each experienced that day. Take it in turns to talk about each emotion and then discuss what you could do to help yourself feel better.

For example:

> *Lola:* Today I felt sad that Daddy was at work – I feel happy when he is at home for bath time.
>
> *Me:* Today I felt worried about you being poorly – I decided to do some mindful breathing to help me relax.

This helps to develop open communication, listening skills and the ability to express ourselves. It gives children an understanding about how to share their emotions. It also demonstrates to children that as adults we also experience feelings and that it's OK to share vulnerabilities.

When children begin to notice that having ups and downs is all part of life it helps reduce their fears and anxieties, and encourages strength, open-ness, trust and companionship.

Faces

Using a whiteboard, blackboard or piece of paper, draw a smiley face on one side of the board or page and a sad face on the other. Continue by talking as a family about how you can turn sad emotions into happier ones and what you can do to help yourself feel better.

Here is an example of what you might write on the whiteboard or paper:

Sad face	Smiley face
To be alone	Share time with friends
To feel tired	Have more sleep to give you more energy
To feel overwhelmed	Be calm and quiet at home
To feel judged	Accept and trust yourself

Tightness in tummy/ anxious	Find time to relax
Sadness	Discover joy in simple things such as nature.

Nature

I have realized that being outside is a key part of my daily routine with Lola and Kit. The fresh air is something we all need and being outdoors is not only important for our health but also for our children's development. Encouraging children to stop, listen and observe their surroundings helps concentration. Outdoor play is a fun way to learn, and spending time outside promotes a healthy lifestyle too. Having an appreciation of nature shows care for our environment.

Being around nature with our children is a creative way to introduce mindfulness into the day too. It teaches a sense of awareness, it engages our senses and gives us the ability to study detail such as colour, texture and smell.

Bringing awareness to sounds, such as the birds, the smell of a flower or touch of the grass under our bare feet, are all calming and gentle reminders to share mindful moments.

Perhaps on my own I wouldn't feel I could take the time to stop and really take in the details of nature, the colours, the sounds, how it smells, how it feels, but when I'm with the children it gives me the perfect excuse to take in the wonder of nature all over again. It is easy to take our surroundings for granted – we've seen different types of flowers, watched the leaves change with the seasons, we've fed the ducks and walked beside a river – but how much do we really take in without our minds wandering or being distracted?

I can take the children to the park and find myself mentally preparing a shopping list, or being distracted by a message on my phone, and before I know it the chance to enjoy a moment of mindfulness with Lola and Kit has passed.

If we observe how a child takes in nature, as if discovering its beauty for the first time, it can be a reminder for us to focus on the present moment, away from our daily distractions, and begin to discover the world around us again through the eyes of a child.

Nature

Here are some short visual and practical exercises to share with the family, using our environment and nature as a way to practise mindfulness. They are engaging, calming and teach the mind to become more focused and present.

Clouds

Lying side by side on the ground, simply watch the clouds go by above you.

Talk about how our mind is like a clear blue sky and each cloud is like a thought.

Like our thoughts, clouds come and go, constantly moving and changing.

This exercise reminds us not to get caught up in thought. It can be used as a visualization during a one-minute mindful practice (see One-minute mindfulness on page 29). When concentrating on our breathing visualize a thought like a cloud and then let it pass by.

I spy

Perfect for a long car journey!

You can use the traditional: 'I spy with my little eye something beginning with C – car.'

With Lola being young I adapt this and use a colour instead of a letter: 'I spy with my little eye something that is green – tree.'

Playing I spy strengthens mindful concentration and brings us into the present moment. It also helps to distract and educate a restless child in the car, even if only for a short time!

Four sticks

While exploring outdoors with your child choose four sticks and place them in a small square on the ground, making a sort of frame. Talk together about the colours and textures of whatever they can see inside the square. The longer you look, the more you can see, so this is a very good exercise to focus attention.

Art

During a walk in the park collect any natural objects you like, such as sticks or fallen leaves, and take them home to create some artwork with. Lola sometimes likes me to take a photo of the flowers we see on our walks so that she can copy and draw them later when we are back at home.

To be fully engaged with a creative project nurtures our ability to get lost in a moment and therefore we are naturally present. Art is one of the first activities children can do that practises mindfulness without realizing it.

Grow a plant

Simply plant a seed and watch your plant grow over the weeks.

Talk about how important it is to care for your plant to help it grow. This demonstrates an understanding of nurturing by remembering to take care of your plant by watering it and giving the plant enough light.

Watching a plant grow is rewarding and gives children confidence and a sense of achievement. It is also a chance to educate them about where our food comes from and why it is important to look after our environment.

This allows us an opportunity to talk about the circle of life and how everything changes and nothing stays the same.

 The garden of your mind

Imagine your mind like a garden. Positive thoughts are the flowers that brighten your life. Negative thoughts are the weeds that spread and get muddled up within the flowers.

Thinking about our emotions like weeds in a garden is a powerful metaphor. Just like our garden, emotions need our attention and must be taken care of. If we ignore how we feel and stop looking after our own well-being, the weeds will grow.

Using this metaphor brings awareness about what helps our own mind thrive and grow rather than becoming tangled and neglected. Which friends are helping you grow and who is bringing challenges to your life?

Looking after yourself is an ongoing process, so when you next look out into a beautiful garden use it as an opportunity to pause and think about how you are, what you need and who it is that makes you shine and flourish.

Simple ways to ease busy lives

Reduce the noise

♡

'Sometimes you've got to to take a break
from all the noise to appreciate the beauty
of the silence.' – Robert Tew

The relationship I have with my phone is something I continue to consider and question daily, as I'm sure many of us do. On the one hand I am grateful for the connection, company and practicality it brings to everyday life, but on the other hand I resent the attention it requires and my dependence on it – I know that I can spend too long attached to a screen. There is also the added guilt of being interrupted by notifications while spending quality time with friends and family, not to mention wanting to set a good example to your children. I know for me when

I'm playing hide-and-seek at the park or simply walking to the shops with Lola chatting away to me, I can begin to feel agitated by the work emails or messages from various family and friend groups that are beeping away at me. I suppose it makes me feel anxious about getting behind or that I'm missing something that requires my attention. The noise around our environment and in our minds becomes busier and louder and our thoughts start to spiral with everything that needs to be done. I'm not saying that we should ignore our phones altogether. I certainly would be lost if I didn't use mine, but I feel better when I try to find a balance.

Technology brings to mind a sense of urgency. We are all so used to instant communication and connection with others that there is an expectation for a quick response and because we are able to connect from anywhere, any time, there is a sense that we are always 'on'. The pressure this puts us all under can be stressful. Social media is part of my job and I realized that it was very important to start setting myself boundaries and learn how best to manage my time spent dedicated to screens. I started to note down the times in the day that I was on my phone (and it was a shock to realize that I was unable to get through a TV programme or go to the loo without it!).

There have been so many positive outcomes to social media and the communities it continues to build. For me it has started many conversations around mental health, fertility and motherhood – big life events that often make people feel lonely because they don't have people who understand what they are going through close to them. Witnessing others openly and honestly talk about topics that in the past could have left you feeling isolated or alone has been incredibly supportive.

Like so many things, positives come with negatives and in this case I reached a point where I felt under pressure to be posting something interesting on social media regularly. This started to dominate too much of my time and often interrupted quality time with family and friends. We're a new generation of social media users, and we are all learning about the impact it has, so I have taken time to consider how to find a balance and to start thinking of ways to use social media and technology as positively as I can and hopefully set an example to Lola and Kit for when they are older.

Since exploring my relationship with screens further I have come to understand more clearly about how it quickly becomes habitual and occasionally addictive. If I am feeling anxious, I tend to reach for my phone, and yet the irony is that the phone can enhance these difficult emotions. If I can't get hold of someone straight away, this can fuel the symptoms of anxiety. If I am feeling overwhelmed or stressed, my phone can often contribute to the mental workload by adding to the list of things to do.

Hopefully with the help of this exercise we can become more mindful about slowing down our pace around technology, encouraging healthier relationships with screens and prioritizing what is urgent, what can wait and, as a result, reduce the noise of technology in our lives. In this exercise I would like to share with you some tips for a healthier relationship with our phones and screens.

Screen boundaries

- It is refreshing to give ourselves permission to walk away from our phones at certain points in the day. Notifications on our phone can fuel anxiety and can quickly pull our focus away from something we are doing or time spent with our family or friends. Allocating moments in the day to turn off notifications until we can give them our full attention is a healthy boundary. That way you have a choice about when to check emails or messages, knowing that not only will you have time to respond, but you will also be able to give them your full attention.

• Consider removing notifications from social media or apps, so that only essential notifications pop up. These alerts add to the daily noise of our phone and it's not always necessary, however much we enjoy the latest gossip from the *Love Island* villa!

• Try putting all social media icons into a separate box on your phone and name it 'Think'. This can remind us to pause and consider whether we really want to spend the time scrolling and also question if it will benefit our current mood or whether we are reaching for it out of habit.

• It might be worth considering which accounts you follow online and asking yourself if they empower and inspire you. I find it helpful to think of my Instagram feed like I'm designing my own magazine, making sure the accounts I follow speak to me positively before engaging with it.

- Have a good clear-out of unwanted emails by unsubscribing from companies you no longer want to receive emails from. One way to make this easier is to create an unsubscribe folder and move unwanted emails here. Then after a week you can set aside time to deal with these all at once.

- Remember to take breaks from looking at the screen. It has been suggested that we should have a break every twenty minutes. There is a rule you can try called 20-20-20, which is that every twenty minutes you take twenty seconds to look at something twenty feet away and stand up and move around if you can. Having a break from the screen gives us the chance to take a step back and recharge, which helps our creativity and productivity.

Reduce the noise

- It is well documented that screens emit a blue light that prevents your body from releasing melatonin, a chemical that helps you sleep. It is suggested that screens be removed two hours before you go to bed. It might be worth considering having a traditional alarm clock by your bed, rather than using the alarm function on your smartphone, meaning you do not need to rely on your phone for the time.

- Decide with your family when during the day to remove screens. Children follow our example, so it's important for them to observe our own screen boundaries.

Mindful ways to use technology

Technology is now very much part of our day-to-day lives and it can also prompt us to be mindful too.

- When the phone rings or a notification pops up use it as a reminder to take a couple of mindful breaths before answering. When your phone rings wait until it has rung at least three times before answering and use each ring as a chance for a mindful breathing cycle (see page 25). This way we can remove ourselves from the mood or situation we have been in and be able to answer calmly and with more focus.

• We can also apply this to when the computer is starting up or while checking our emails. It has been suggested that we naturally hold our breath when reading or writing emails. Next time you read or write an email bring your awareness to breathing and take two full mindful breaths before replying. It may take a little extra time but your mind will be clearer and more peaceful as a result, therefore giving your thoughts more clarity.

• Set reminders on your phone for a quick time out to practise one minute of mindfulness (see page 29) or you could do an exercise from this book.

- Be mindful about when you reach for your phone and ask yourself if it is out of boredom? Perhaps this is a reminder to allow yourself to be in a space of nothing for a moment, with no screen, giving yourself permission to set your imagination free!

Multitasking

♡

Multitasking is one of the main culprits for taking away our ability to live mindfully. How can we be fully engaged with life emotionally and physically when we are doing three jobs at once and overstimulating ourselves?

As mums we put ourselves under so much pressure, not just about all the things we feel we should be doing for our family but also the pressure to get everything on the to-do list done and to get it right! As household jobs pile up we can find ourselves becoming flustered by the simplest tasks, such as unloading a dishwasher, keeping on top of the washing, making breakfast or preparing a packed lunch, all of which we are trying to complete at once!

My multitasking is at its craziest during the children's teatime; I'm determined to get as many jobs done as I can so that once the children are in bed I can have some time for myself – not surrounded by toys, a pile of washing-up and a basket full of clothes that need folding. However, I have found that I can be more productive and use my time more efficiently once the children are in bed and actually get the jobs done in peace, in less time and without a little one hanging off my leg.

Being mindful about this gives us the chance to pay attention to the moment and also helps remind us to stop and take each task one at a time, which can feel less stressful. Learning to prioritize what needs our attention and what can wait is also vital for our own peace of mind.

My five top tips to help bring awareness to multi-tasking:

1. Write a list of the most important tasks that need completing and work through them in order.

2. Avoid being distracted by your phone while in the middle of an activity.

3. Don't be afraid to say no if you have too many tasks to complete already that day.

4. Start to pay attention and be aware of your multitasking habits.

5. Finish one task before moving on to the next.

Autopilot awareness

♡

We are all creatures of habit, so living on autopilot is a natural response to the repetition of our daily lives. However, this can often allow us to avoid how we really feel emotionally, and our awareness can become hazy.

How many times have you taken a journey and when you arrive wonder how you got there because you can't remember anything distinctive about it? Or mentally gone through your to-do list while taking part in a completely different activity? Even very small changes, like changing the mug we drink from every morning, adding something new to the weekly food shop, wearing something that you thought you would save for a special occasion, these all help us break the habits of being on autopilot.

It is natural to multitask and live on autopilot, especially around the monotony of our children's routines. As mums, living on autopilot is something we do every day to help us stay on top of the daily mental load. It may seem to help us feel in control but learning to let go and embrace change can help free us from stress and anxiety.

Using the tips below is a helpful way to teach us to notice these automatic responses and to begin to change our thought processes.

- Be present and focus on each activity individually. Staying mindful helps us remove the urge to start a new activity and allows our attention to remain focused on the task we are completing.

- Take on one activity at a time and ask yourself whether it could wait.

- Turn off notifications on your phone to prevent interruptions and set aside times in the day to check emails and messages.

- Choose your daily activities wisely and question whether you are taking on too much.

- Plan your day and try something new, like a different route to work or school.

- Be observant about your surroundings, even if it's a space you have been in many times. Look for something new that you haven't noticed before.

- When using your phone to take photos use it as a chance to really take in all the detail of the photograph.

- When the children are in bed take some time to organize what you can for the next day so that the following morning doesn't feel so hectic.

- Think about what time of day you feel most productive and plan your day accordingly.

Perspective in motherhood

♡

Gaining perspective is something that usually happens when we are faced with difficulty. We have all had those wake-up calls, forcing us to slow down and realize what is important. It is during these moments we think about putting our lives into perspective. This could be anything from illness or a breakdown in a relationship, right through to the challenges we face in motherhood.

If you are sitting at home with your baby, who, for example, is refusing a nap or is unwell, or perhaps a toddler learning to potty-train or having a meltdown, it can feel very frustrating, demanding and lonely. It is all-consuming, and in that moment it feels like the most important thing. We are understandably consumed by these emotions and can quickly lose a sense of perspective.

I relate to this most when I think about when I was potty-training Lola. We were stuck in the house for a week and it felt like I was going slowly mad. I was unable to be rational about the situation. I lost all sense of perspective and any connection with what was going on outside. The levels of frustration built up each time we missed the potty, knowing it was going to be a good few hours before we had the chance to try again! I blamed myself, feeling like I was getting it wrong or somehow letting Lola down. The irony of this was that actually when we eventually left the house and got on with living our life as normal, I relaxed and therefore Lola did too. Stepping out of the situation helped me gain perspective and reminded me to think about the bigger picture.

Here is a simple exercise you can use to think about gaining perspective. You can practise this exercise with your eyes open or closed.

- Imagine you are using your thumb and first finger (as you would on a phone screen) to slowly zoom out of a challenging situation.

- Visualize what is happening
  outside of the moment you are in.

- Visualize yourself and the situation
  you are in becoming smaller and
  smaller when looking at the bigger
  picture from above.

For example, if you're at home, start with visualizing the room you are in, then your house, then the street where you live, gradually expanding into the town and beyond. It is up to you how detailed you are with all you can see. Imagine daily life continuing around you, and as you mentally zoom out you could think of the mantra 'This too shall pass'.

Hopefully this will help you to find perspective and for you to feel less trapped by the situation and emotion you are experiencing in that moment.

It is completely natural to bring up our children to feel that they are the centre of our universe because we love them so much, but over time we also need to bring perspective into their lives, so this is a great exercise to share with your children as they get older.

Slowing down

♡

'Life's rich tapestry.'

On many occasions growing up my dad would say these words to me, but until recently I never thought about their true meaning.

If we really think about this, we can start to imagine all the individual colourful woven threads entwining with each other and slowly creating the bigger picture of our lives. Taking a step back and picturing ourselves at the end of our life, looking at our tapestry, what would we want to see . . . ? What has been most meaningful to you, most important and when have you felt at your happiest?

When you think about happy memories, per- haps times with your family and friends, being on holiday, enjoying your hobbies and interests, it's most likely that these have been times when your pace of life has been slower and you have naturally been living more mindfully.

I've often wondered what would happen if we took away the clock. As a mum I have become so aware of all that needs to be done by a certain time. We are dictated to by our children's routines and time can feel like an added pressure to the busyness of our day-to-day lives, especially when we are try-ing to meet deadlines of our own.

The trouble is that we often pride ourselves on being busy, trying to cram as much as we can into as little time as possible. Of course, there are times when living at a faster pace is appropriate and the exhilaration can feel exciting. However, constantly living in this state can be a distraction from how we truly feel emotionally and physically.

We might think that slowing down is lazy or per-haps we thrive on the buzz of adrenaline, thinking that being busy means we are achieving more – always in a hurry to move on to the next activity instead of simply being where we are right now.

If we step back and notice that we actually find more enjoyment from life when we slow down, this is usually because we have the time to take in the joy that surrounds us, so even though being busy has its place it shouldn't be our constant way of living.

Here are a few reminders to help us think about slowing down:

- Try to consciously notice when you are rushing through life instead of truly living it.

- Take the time to connect with the moment and person you are with.

- Stick to one activity at a time and remain fully present.

- When you are hurrying through your day ask yourself, what is most important to me today?

- Practise a mindful exercise as a reminder to slow down and create space in your day.

- Be mindful about keeping perspective (see Perspective in motherhood on page 197), have an awareness about being on autopilot, and observe how much time you spend multitasking.

- So often we live for tomorrow; however, one day we will look back and long for today.

Truly listening

♡

'The art of listening is a wonderful gift.'

This exercise is about taking the time to really listen to one another. This could mean listening to a family member, child, friend or work colleague. If we are able to listen properly, not only are we helping others but it also enables us to manage difficult situations, emotions, disagreements or issues in a calm manner, remembering to avoid judgement or the need to fill a silence with your experience and opinions. It is natural to want to try to help, to try to fix things for people, to make everything better, but sometimes people want nothing more than the simple action of being listened to. Being heard is sometimes enough and something we all need from time to time.

Noticing when someone would like to be listened to, including our children, is often the first step. I've noticed that Lola might choose to share an emotion with me, usually while I'm busy trying to complete another task or rushing out of the house for an appointment. If we allow the moment to pass, it might be that they don't give us another opportunity to listen to what they are trying to say. Of course, Lola is still young, but the type of thing she might say is 'I feel sad today because my friend didn't want to play with me' or 'I miss Daddy', but then she quickly moves on to the next activity. As she grows these emotions will develop, I'm sure, so I'm trying to practise with the help of this listening exercise to keep the lines of communication open so that for the bigger stuff Lola knows I'm always here to listen.

With Harry and I it is all about finding the right moment to talk, a time when we can both listen to one another. We have had to work on this a lot since having children as it is often hard to find the right time and space. I find it very difficult to concentrate on conversations when Lola and Kit are around; naturally, there is more noise and demands, so it's not always easy to focus and give one another attention. While Harry is talking it is also very possible for my mind to be running ahead, thinking about what needs preparing for dinner, a bill that needs paying and the wash that needs to go into the tumble dryer! Equally, at the end of the day, once Lola and Kit are in bed, I find I need a little time to unwind and quieten my busy mind before having the energy and brain power to focus.

Harry and I have worked out that the best time for us to talk is often over dinner. We have recently moved house so there has been lots of admin to discuss and organize along with conversations about where we should live, the children's education, etc. We know that discussing these heavy topics in front of the children during a trip to the park or bath time is not the optimum moment, however tempting. We soon realized that a conversation that had been going on in short snippets over two weeks of trying to snatch moments here and there could have been resolved more quickly had we dedicated listening time for it.

Here is an exercise about listening, and although it might seem quite formal, it can really help the other person to feel they have the time and space to talk and be heard. You can adapt the wording to suit the situation but this gives you an idea about how the exercise works:

- Begin by making sure you are in a
  safe and comfortable place to be
  able to listen without distraction.

- Tell the person you are with that
  they have your full attention to
  listen to their worries and concerns.

- When they start talking allow
  them to say all they need to
  without interruption.

- Once they have finished speaking
  ask if there is anything else they
  would like to share.

- Once the person has finished
  talking continue by summarizing
  their words. It's important not to
  add your own opinions or
  experiences or to try to fix anything.

- Finish by saying 'Have I heard
  what you've said correctly?' and
  'Is there anything you would like
  to add?'

Opening up emotionally is not something we all
find easy. We might prefer to avoid confrontation

or feel we don't have the energy for disagreement. Life is busy and time is precious, so perhaps we feel guilty for taking up other people's time talking about ourselves or find it difficult to trust others with our emotions. We might question if what we want to say is important enough, assuming our worries will be small in comparison to other people's. However big or small, we should all feel able to lighten the load, be listened to and, more importantly, heard.

Spread a little happiness

Sharing mindful moments with your family

'Any day spent with you is my favourite day.
So, today is my new favourite day.'
– A. A. Milne, *Winnie-the-Pooh*

Mindfulness improves our overall sense of well-being and helps us to relax the mind and body. This section includes mindful activities to share with your children and for you to enjoy. Each of these exercises aims to focus your mind on the present, allowing you to slow down and enjoy the moment together.

A wall of love

Write the word 'LOVE' big enough that you can cut out each letter and stick it to a wall in your house.

Using notes (we like to cut out heart shapes) write a message to stick around the word 'love' and watch your family love wall grow.

- 'I love my mum because she gives the best cuddles.'
- 'I love spending time playing games together.'
- 'I love dancing to music.'
- 'I love sharing an ice cream with Granny.'
- 'I love having my friends over for tea.'
- 'I love watching a film together.'
- 'I love peanut butter.'

This wall can be added to any time you like when you want to express yourself about something you love and that makes you happy.

A memory book

With your children, choose photos to print, including moments you've shared with anyone you love. This could include places you've visited or activities you have enjoyed. Because all my photos are stored on my phone, I often don't print photos like I used to, but to have a keepsake like a memory book is a very special gift to treasure as a family. Remembering happy times can help to elevate your mood, which I have found helpful when feeling anxious.

It is also an opportunity to share photos of our past generations who may no longer be with us, but who you would like your children to learn more about. I was very close to my granny so I would like Lola and Kit to know what she looked like and for me to have the chance to tell them all about her and the happy memories we shared. Lola often still talks about our cat Murphy who passed away and how 'Murphy has gone to the sky'. I find the memory book a useful opportunity to talk about the circle of life.

It needn't just be a book of those we have lost. Harry's sister and her family live in Singapore, so we don't see them as often as we would like and having a memory book means we can talk about them too and about the happy holidays we have shared together.

It is a lovely activity at bedtime to look through your memory book, as it is comforting to talk about those we love and the times that have made us smile. These are good emotions to feel before going to bed and with your children you can send well wishes to your loved ones before going to sleep.

Creating a memory book is a beautiful way to keep your memories alive and it will be something you can continue to add to, cherish and look back on over the years.

Music playlist

Music is a huge part of my family's life, so we like to create playlists together. It is something we all enjoy doing and we talk about why each song means something special to us.

On the Judds' playlist, you can find songs like: The Beach Boys' 'Don't Worry Baby', which was playing when Harry proposed; Michael Bublé's version of 'Can't Help Falling in Love', which was our first wedding dance; and Lola and Kit's favourite from Daddy's band McFly, 'Love is on the Radio'.

Music makes us all feel good, so listening to playlists can be helpful for those fractious tired moments or for keeping us energized and entertained during a long car journey. It is a fun activity to create together and children love to listen to their own playlists!

Colouring

Colouring is one of my favourite activities to share with Lola and Kit. As a family, this is something we all find satisfying and rewarding, especially when we have each finished our masterpiece artwork!

Everyone needs a calm moment and a chance to wind down, including children. Colouring is naturally a mindful activity and a great way to teach and bring mindfulness into our children's day. Colouring together encourages us to sit down and concentrate on one activity. It wakes up our senses and focuses our minds. It gives us all the chance to take a breather, quieten down and find the calm in the business of the day. It helps reduce stress, improve mood, concentration and focus, and for young children it also helps develop fine motor skills. A colouring book and pencils are now a staple in my bag and have come to the rescue on many occasions, mainly in restaurants (until Peppa Pig makes an appearance!).

I struggle with what to do with all the children's artwork so have started a scrapbook with my favourites, and then we also use some to put in birthday cards or to send as a little gesture to let grandparents or friends know we are thinking of them.

Using the prompts below can help to keep our attention on the present moment when our mind starts wandering.

The following example is for a young child but the idea can be adapted for any age.

How can I use colouring to practise mindfulness?

1. Start by asking what the picture is that you are colouring and what details can you see?

   For example, in this picture I see a teddy bear holding an umbrella. He is wearing wellington boots and a raincoat. The teddy bear is standing in a puddle and there are raindrops splashing on the umbrella.

2. Then ask what colours shall we use?

   For example, blue for the raindrops, red for the wellington boots, and yellow for the raincoat.

3. At this point we can begin to talk about how the teddy bear might be feeling. He has a smile on his face so he looks happy to be in the rain. The umbrella is keeping him dry and it looks like the puddle has a few splashes, so he must have had fun jumping up and down in it.

4. As we begin colouring we can move our attention to our senses, starting with the motion of our hand, the way our fingers hold the pencil and how our hand is moving. Is the pressure on the page light or hard? What sound can you hear as the pencil moves across the page? Then there is the smell of a freshly sharpened pencil, which always reminds me of being at school and the smell of my pencil case!

Music

I met Harry on McFly's Wonderland arena tour in 2005. I was booked to play the violin as part of the backing orchestra and I can honestly say the first time I looked at Harry it was love at first sight. It was also during this tour that I met the other girls from Escala.

Having met Harry through music, you can imagine how important it is to us both for music to be part of our family's life. Having grown up surrounded by music, I want to include music in our day-to-day life. Not only do I find playing my violin and music to my children engaging and relaxing, it is also a useful way to change the mood or distract squabbling siblings! I also sing my way through most activities and have made up songs to get through the simplest tasks that somehow with children become stressful, such as putting on sun cream, getting dressed, changing a nappy, encouraging them to eat vegetables, washing hair, trying to leave the house, putting on shoes (the list goes on!), but also for calmer moments, such as a lullaby at bedtime or during a happy walk outside.

Singing changes the tone of our voice and stimulates a different response and atmosphere for both you and the children. It really doesn't matter how your voice sounds or if you can or can't sing, your children will always enjoy listening to you sing to them.

As a baby develops in the womb the only one of our senses that fully develops is hearing. Therefore the sound of a mother's voice is one of a baby's first sensory experiences. Research has shown that the maternal voice plays a direct role in hearing and language development. During both my pregnancies I played music through special headphones that I placed on my bump. I was amazed after Lola was born that listening to the music I had played to her in the womb noticeably soothed her. For Kit it was the sound of Harry practising on his drum pad night after night on the sofa next to me in my pregnancy! I suppose the rhythmic pattern is like white noise and to this day Kit is calmed by this sound. Me, not so much!

When Lola was a baby we were keen to find a local music class, so we started going to Monkey Music when she was just four months old. I remember our first class and feeling very much in that newborn hormonal foggy bubble. At that stage leaving the house was an achievement, and I constantly felt nervous about Lola needing a feed or what to do if she cried, especially during a baby class. Of course I didn't need to worry, because I was surrounded by others with the same fears and babies that cried too! Both Lola and I quickly made friends with the others in the class and it became something we looked forward to each week. I could see music was helping with her development and through these early years watching the simple joy on both Lola and Kit's faces through music has been magical.

Music teaches us skills that we will continue to use whatever career we end up in. The ability to work as a team, an understanding about discipline, the ability to communicate, sheer hard work and proof that life takes practice.

When thinking about music and mindfulness I have realized just how much the two are connected. Mainly because in music, like in mindfulness, we use our senses such as sight, hearing and touch; it also requires complete focus to learn an instrument, all of which encourages our mind to remain present.

Sharing mindful moments with your family

Here is a simple way to learn mindfulness through music with young children:

- Using musical instruments, such as rattles, shakers, drums or any toy that makes a sound, encourage children to concentrate on their senses.

- Talk about what they can hear and, while listening to a nursery rhyme, play along with the different instruments. Does the rattle sound like a bell?

- Talk about all the different colours they can see on the instruments. Perhaps the shaker has lots of colours like a rainbow.

- Talk about what it feels like to play the drum. To make a loud sound we tap harder and for quieter sounds we tap the drum softly.

An exercise for you

Begin this exercise by choosing some simple music without too much emotion attached to it. This could be classical music or meditation music with a slower tempo.

Music often brings up different emotions so it's important the music you choose doesn't encourage your mind to wander off into happy or sad nostalgia.

- Find a comfortable and quiet place to sit and gently close your eyes.

- Soften the muscles in your face and allow your body to relax.

- Listen to the music with all your attention; perhaps you haven't listened with as much detail before or heard all the different instruments being played.

- If your mind wanders, bring your attention back to the music.

- Breathe.

Mindful story time

Reading with children is a very beneficial mindful practice that includes many health benefits, such as reducing stress, relaxation and increasing our knowledge. I also find it pleasant to enjoy a traditional form of entertainment that takes our eyes away from screens. Reading is something that can be shared together as a family.

Storytelling goes back thousands of years and is still very much part of our lives. Stories allow us to look at the world with a different perspective, and they improve our understanding about compassion and empathy, while also teaching the importance of morals and values. Reading is fun and relaxing for children, while also supporting emotional and cognitive development. It connects children to the world around them, captivating their attention and creativity while also sparking imaginations.

Reading with children allows a safe space to talk about the different emotions that your child might relate to in the book.

My favourite example of this is Winnie-the-Pooh. If we look at the individual characters and all they represent, we can relate whatever age we are.

Winnie-the-Pooh, a caring loyal friend; Piglet, who tries so hard to be brave; Tigger, who is playful and childish; Kanga, the kind and understanding mother; Rabbit, who has all the best intentions but is short-tempered and fussy; Owl, who is wise; and Roo, who is clever and adventurous.

Mindful reading is something we can practise daily while reading to our children. I can easily switch into autopilot, not really taking in what I'm reading about. My mind wanders off, especially when reading books at bedtime when I'm often hungry and too tired to concentrate, so I begin to think about what I'm going to cook for dinner or about running myself a bath!

To combat this I've started to include reading books to Lola and Kit at other times in the day, such as first thing in the morning or during the afternoon when we are perhaps in need of sharing a quieter moment together.

Here are a few tips for mindful reading with your children:

- Create a space that is quiet with few distractions.

- Try not to get stuck with the same books; a trip to the library is a calm outing for you and your children, and you can enjoy quiet story time there too.

- Connect with your inner child and share the excitement of a story as if reading it for the first time.

- Really listen to the words and engage with the pictures.

- Have fun with giving each character a different voice.

- Go on the adventure with your child.

- Read slowly to give yourself the chance to take the moment in.

- At the end of each day, before putting the children to bed, this is a way to unwind together, put any worries of the day behind you and share a peaceful moment (unless a toddler has other plans, in which case just try again the next night!).

family list

The heart of this exercise is to bring awareness to the needs of each member of the family, making sure that the things that are important to each person are recognized by the others. It is good to look after one another and it helps day-to-day family life run so much more smoothly too. Discovering what makes each member of the family happy and sharing these with one another is a fun exercise to do together at the start of each month.

As a family create a list of what is important for you all individually but also some activities you enjoy doing together. This also helps to plan ahead for the days you have as a family.

This gives children the chance to talk about what they do and don't enjoy doing. It allows us to discuss and bring awareness to daily chores that need completing in a positive light, showing team effort and encouraging self-discipline. It also demonstrates to children that parents have their own interests and hobbies.

How to create your family list:

- Find an area in your house where you can write down your individual and family lists for the month. This could be on a noticeboard or whiteboard or a piece of paper you stick to the fridge.

- As activities are completed mark with a heart for each member of the family to see and check that everyone's needs are being met.

- Discuss responsibilities, such as helping make the beds, brushing teeth, getting school bags ready, helping with the recycling, putting the shopping away and tidying bedrooms.

Family list

Examples that work
for our family:

Mum:

An hour in the house to myself.

A bath.

Dinner with friends.

Exercise.

Going to the cinema with Daddy.

Dad:

Watch sport on the TV.

Go to the gym.

Time with friends.

Playing cricket or golf.

Lola and Kit:

Go to the park.

Play a game together.

Play date with friends.

Colouring.

Play-Doh.

Time alone with Mummy
and Daddy.

Family:

Listen to how everyone else's
day was.

Clear up together.

Read books.

Water the garden.

Make the beds.

Listen to music together.

Plan a day trip.

Bike ride.

Kindness

♡

'In a world where you can be anything,
be kind.' – Jennifer Dukes Lee

It is often the smallest acts of kindness that are most rewarding. A smile, a kind word, taking the time to listen, opening the door for a stranger. Whatever it might be, kindness strengthens relationships and will always make the world a better place.

Thinking about kindness daily within mother-hood is key. We often question our actions, constantly asking ourselves if we're doing a good enough job, with high expectations adding even more volume to the noise in our minds.

I am guilty of speaking unkindly to myself, with a little critic who sits on my shoulder and talks to me about all sorts of negative things, and generally questioning if I'm being a good enough mum, perhaps thinking that others seem to be doing a better job and that I'm somehow letting my children down. I've realized I rarely say anything kind to myself, like it was wonderful to play my violin to Lola and Kit today or about the time we spent colouring or the fact they have food in their tummies!

I'm often in a boxing ring with myself, but what if I choose to leave that unkind voice behind? One of the most important acts of self-care is to remember to speak kindly.

There are many ways to practise and share kindness daily. Here are a few exercises that you might find helpful.

Speak kindly

I find it increasingly tough to remain calm when my children are pushing my buttons and I don't like the sound of my voice if I become impatient, but, as we all know, when it's been a long day or a long night and we're running low on energy we often say things we don't mean.

When bringing awareness to kindness in these moments try to think about making a choice to speak and think kindly. I've noticed that in these challenging moments when it feels like no one is listening, if I change my language from words of frustration to words of kindness, this can help me handle emotions more positively and in return I receive a calmer response from my children (and my husband!).

Taking the time for kindness

This is a simple mindful exercise to help you take notice when someone is being kind to you and when you can be kind to others.

How do we take the time to be kind?

- Talk.

- Listen without judgement.

- Smile.

- Help and support.

- Be ourselves and let others be themselves.

- Let others know they are not alone.
- Let someone know you are thinking of them.
- Hug.
- Be there.
- Give someone your time.
- Ask if you're OK.
- Find time for yourself.
- Tell someone they are doing a great job.
- Give a compliment.
- Remind others to be kind to themselves.
- Slow down.
- Check in and say hi – being a new mum can be lonely.

Kindness jar

This is so simple, but effective in reminding us all about being kind.

All you need is a jar, some marbles or paper and a pen that can decorate the glass jar.

With your child talk about how it feels when someone is kind to them and how important it is to spread kindness to others around them and at home. When you or your child does something kind for someone else, as a family you can put a marble into the jar, or, if you would prefer, write a note about the act of kindness and put it inside the jar.

For example:

- I am kind when I write a card for a friend who is feeling sad.

- I am kind when I clean up my toys without being asked.

- I am kind when I ask a friend how they are.

- I am kind when I set the table for dinner.

- I am kind when I let my brother choose our bedtime story.

Watching the jar fill up is rewarding and keeps the conversation going about kindness and thinking of others.

Random acts of kindness

Here are a couple of ideas about random acts of kindness that help bring joy to others:

- Write a letter to someone who has made an impact on your life in some way. Perhaps a teacher or adult who supported you growing up. For your children this could be a teacher or friend who has done something kind for them.

  A simple note to say thank you would mean so much to that person. It is a cathartic exercise for an adult and a good lesson for our children to remember to thank others and to begin noticing when

someone has shown kindness
to them.

- For a younger child to draw or
paint something to send to a
family member.

Lola's grandfather was recently
home alone for two weeks because
her granny was away visiting
Harry's sister. Lola sent a painting
and we included a note saying 'We
hope you are not too lonely with
Granny away and that this painting
makes you smile.'

Going through the process of
posting the letter gave Lola
responsibility and an awareness
about thinking of others, and her
grandfather was touched to
receive it.

Set a kindness intention

Talk with your child about an act of kindness that
they can set as an intention for that day.

For example:

- Hold the door open for someone.
- Put some clothes away.
- Share a special toy with a friend.

Speaking kindness

Something I have become more aware of since becoming a mum is the way I talk to myself and the language I use in front of Lola and Kit. I feel a responsibility to speak with honesty, while also keeping an awareness about the impact my words could have on their own thought patterns.

This is something I also consider when it comes to body image. After having children our bodies inevitably change. Remembering to appreciate and respect our bodies takes practice. This exercise aims to help build self-confidence and to encourage friendly language. This can help both you and your child even if you feel a little bit awkward at first!

With your child look in the mirror and invite them to say something kind or something they like about themselves. Lola might say 'I like my curly hair' or 'I'm happy when I'm dancing'. Next I will do the same. I'll say something like 'I like my hands because they let me play the violin'.

How many times have you stood in front of the mirror and thought something kind about your reflection or even smiled at your reflection?

I hope introducing this exercise at a young age will help Lola and Kit to speak and think kindly about themselves and encourage a healthy confidence.

Charge up your hearts

♡♡

Starting nursery or school is a huge milestone for all the family. I remember on Lola's first day at nursery feeling like she was starting a new adventure, but this time without me there to protect her. I was nervous, sad and excited all at once! It was the realization that she was becoming her own little person and that I would need to trust others to take care of her and inspire her. What if someone was unkind, what if she needed help with something and the teachers didn't notice, what if she didn't settle, what if she cried and started looking for me? I left the nursery that day with a glaze of tears in my eyes that stayed for the rest of the day.

Even though I knew Lola was in safe hands in a

creative and caring environment where she would have the space to grow, make new friends and build confidence, I couldn't help but find it hard to take the first step in letting her go – letting go of control and the need to nurture and protect her. Though I understood that this was a natural and important progression for us both and I also knew in time we would both settle into our new routine.

To ease my worries I wanted to find something that would comfort us both during this transition and came across this exercise.

Drawing a heart on the palm of your hand and the palm of your child's hand, you can explain to your child that when they feel sad they can press the heart to feel a hug from you.

- Draw a heart on the palm of your hand and on the palm of your child's hand.

- Holding hands on the way to school, explain that we are charging up our hearts.

- Then explain that during the day if they are feeling worried, upset or

just in need of some comfort and
reassurance, they can press the
heart on the palm of their hand
to charge up their heart and feel
a hug from you.

Another idea to use for yourself is to add an
affirmation to this exercise so that each time you
are feeling a difficult emotion about settling your
child into school or nursery you can use the heart
as a mindfulness reminder to be gentle on yourself
and stay positive.

- I can take things one day at a time.
- This feeling will pass.
- Today will be a good day.
- Everything will be OK.
- I breathe in confidence and release
  all fears.

Gratitude

'It is not happiness that makes us grateful
but gratefulness that makes us happy.'
– David Steindl-Rast

It is very easy for days to fly past without seeing all
we have to be thankful for; perhaps we spend more
time focusing on what we wish we did have. I can
get so caught up in the rhythm of my day, with many
days feeling repetitive, that I forget to notice the
small things that actually make a big difference to my
overall happiness.

Do I live at such a pace that maybe I don't see
the small gestures of kindness, too wrapped up in
getting from A to B and rushing against the clock?
It's the little things that perhaps go unnoticed that

we would miss if they weren't there any more. The quick phone call to my mum in the morning to check in with each other, the shop assistant who waves hello and smiles at Lola and Kit on our walk to nursery, my local library that gives me the space to work quietly. When you stop to think about it there are endless things to be grateful for if we give ourselves a chance to see them.

Why gratitude?

It is thought that people who practise gratitude are likely to sleep better, feel more positive, more respectful, less materialistic, less stressed, have increased self-esteem, are more optimistic and patient, are more likely to help others, have well-balanced blood pressure and a greater sense of happiness. Gratitude also helps to strengthen relationships and improves overall health and well-being.

When we are stuck in the cycle of daily routines it is easy to take the little things for granted. I often focus on the things that went wrong rather than being grateful for what went right. Using a gratitude practice each day is a way of reminding us what we are thankful for and helps us to change negative thinking into positive thinking. Here are some ideas about how to practise gratitude for you and the family.

Letters

I was recently invited for lunch at a neighbour's house. She had moved to the area after her husband had passed away suddenly. In the kitchen she had a pinboard filled with letters and notes that they had written to one another over the years. It made me realize just how important it is to write to our loved ones; seeing handwriting and reading words of love is irreplaceable. Similarly when I recently opened one of my first ever books, *The Blue Balloon* by Mick Inkpen, to read to Lola and Kit I noticed my grandmother's handwriting in the front. It moved me to tears to see it and see the words 'From Granny, 1989'.

As a child, every Christmas and birthday, I remember sitting down with my brothers to write thank-you letters. Over the years and since technology has become such a quick and easy route to make contact I have found myself writing letters less and less, but another way of writing down gratitude could be to leave notes around the house for your loved ones to find and read.

So, this is a little challenge to get writing – perhaps write to someone you love or to someone you are grateful for once a month. We all know how happy it makes us to receive a handwritten letter in the post!

Gratitude message

Invite a friend or family member to send you a gratitude message at the end of each day for a week. I recently shared this with one of my friends. We are really close and message often, but until we started sending each other messages about the things we've been grateful for each day, I realized I didn't know what her day looked like or what was going on in her life. The things we share with one another won't necessarily have anything to do with the other. I might share things about Harry and the children, but by having agreed to do it daily it encourages us both to take the time to acknowledge what we have been thankful for. It also builds trust between us as sometimes the things we are grateful for are quite small but they could be quite revealing. We've learned a lot about one another and we've also found that it opens the door for us to talk about our feelings, whereas previously when we asked each other how we were the answer might be 'OK, thanks,' even on the days when we really weren't OK at all.

For example:

- Today I'm grateful for our home – having thought about leaving the area and deciding to stay, it has made me realize how happy we are here.

- *Today I was grateful to be in the car for a few hours with my husband. No phones out, no iPads or TV. It gave us a chance to talk about plans and dreams for our family, without having the distractions of technology.*

- Today I'm grateful for so many activities for toddlers where we live, especially the fun gym class that has such a lovely teacher. The girls love it and I can have some time chatting to other mums.

- *Today I was grateful for my friend picking my son up from school. I had huge mum guilt being at work and she made it so much easier by sending me videos of him walking out of the school with a smile and then playing so happily with her girls. It felt so right because I knew he felt secure.*

- Today I was grateful for time with Lola, just the two of us.

- *Today I was grateful that my mum reassured me that my daughter would be OK and comforted me when my baby was crying for me. She made me feel secure in my parenting when I really questioned it, which helped me carry on my day without worrying.*

- Today I was grateful for spending time at my parents' house with Lola and Kit. I loved watching my dad making them laugh and seeing Lola holding my mum's hand and playing with her wedding rings the way I remember doing when I was younger.

- *Today I was grateful to be there at the right moment to give my friend a big cuddle.*

- Today I was grateful for Harry making the bed . . . Sometimes it's the little things!

- *I was so grateful for my wonderful sister who drove up to see my daughter. She was so excited and it was a great distraction from the stressful week and me going away, which I felt anxious about.*

- Today I was grateful for a lovely dinner out with friends. I love spending time with my children, but sharing laughter with other women lifts my spirits up so much.

- *Today I am grateful for my little family. Spending time all together is what I treasure most. With my hubby being away each week it can be tough on me and the girls, so I live for the weekends and our quality time as a family.*

Gratitude journal

Writing a gratitude journal means we can keep a record of all the things we are thankful for and keep track of the positives in our lives. Having a daily recap is a therapeutic and calm way to start and end each day. Writing encourages us to be mindful as we focus our attention on our thoughts, and it also gives us the opportunity to express ourselves in a way that we might find difficult to do openly with others.

For example, start your morning by noting down three things you are grateful for about the day ahead.

- I am grateful that I can work from home.
- I am grateful for sunshine.
- I am grateful for my family's support.

This could also include a moment to observe the simple things we are grateful for in our own home – imagine not having a fridge, a washing machine, heating?

At the end of the day, when perhaps you have more time, you could write down in more detail some thoughts about your day. Here is an example from my gratitude journal:

'Waking up in a comfy bed at home with my family. A nourishing breakfast. The nursery teachers who took care of Lola and Kit so I could work. The girl at the coffee shop who smiled, said hello and made me a coffee. The books I read to educate and inspire me. The food delivery to my door saving me a trip with a tired toddler to the supermarket. Technology that helped me be creative. My phone that let me speak to my mum. The doctor who checked Kit's sore toe! Listening and dancing to music with Lola and Kit. Harry cooking dinner. Putting my feet up and watching TV with my cat, and to my friend who gave me a lavender pillow spray to help me sleep well . . .'

Another idea to include in your journal is to spend sixty seconds thinking about when someone did something kind for you. You can then note down how that made you feel and how you could do something similar for someone else.

Jar of hearts (a gratitude journal
option for children)

This exercise helps share gratitude and kindness with your children. All you need is an empty glass jar and some paper.

- Cut the paper into different shapes, such as hearts or stars. Each day ask your child what they have been thankful for or what they did to be kind to someone?

- Write the short message or word on the paper and start collecting your notes in the jar.

A gratitude stone

Choose a stone with your family, perhaps a pebble from a beach that you brought home from a holiday. At dinner time hand the stone around to each member of the family and as each person takes it they share something they have been grateful for that day.

Gratitude drawings

Younger children may not yet be able to write down their gratitude, so drawing can be a creative and fun way to express themselves. It is a way of teaching what being grateful means and children feel a sense of achievement showing you their art-work. You can share this exercise together; here are some suggestions:

Draw something . . .

- That makes you happy.
- That helps you feel better.
- That makes you smile.
- That you love.
- That you think is fun.
- That makes you laugh.

Gratitude tree

This is a lovely activity for a rainy day at home!
With a large sheet of paper begin by drawing a

tree with empty branches. You can either continue this activity at a table or stick the paper to a wall in your home close to the ground for little people to reach.

Using notes or cut-outs of leaf-shaped paper, begin sticking words of gratitude to the branches of your tree. For example, 'family', 'teachers', 'books', 'music', 'friends', 'kindness', etc.

With your children you can count all you are grateful for, talk about your appreciation for the little things and see all the positives that help us to flourish and grow just like the gratitude tree.

A more permanent fixture in your home could be to have a vase with some sticks or small branches in it. You could hang notes of gratitude off it with ribbon. You can keep adding to your gratitude tree over time.

A family gratitude book

Teaching our children about gratitude gives them the skills to be thoughtful and is also a respectful reminder about treating others how we would like to be treated. It is important not only to express our gratitude through words but also through our actions.

Having a family gratitude book is a lovely keep-sake. Within the book create sections, one for each member of the family; you could personalize the book by having a photo of each family member at the front of each section. Then whenever you choose, you each write down what you have been thankful to the other members of your family for, noting them down in their section. This encourages appreciation for one another and is a wonderful way to help your children know how much they matter – and yourself for that matter! This gives us a sense of belonging and encourages compassion and confidence.

'The best way to show my gratitude is
to accept everything, even my problems,
with joy.' – Mother Teresa

A final thought...

'Ignore the noise,
and the silence will be golden.'

I wrote *Mindfulness for Mums* for anyone who, like me,
might feel as if they have been thrown in at the deep
end of motherhood and are looking for ways to find
balance and calm in their daily lives.

Being a mum is the most powerful experience
emotionally and yet trying to find our flow, learning to let go and finding joy in parenting requires
work and our attention.

Allowing the time for space and reflection
through our mindful practice opens up the opportunity to be compassionate and gentle with ourselves

and in return we are able to share a more mindful way of living with our family, a skill which will continue to benefit not only our lives but also the lives of our children.

I hope with the help of the exercises from this book you will acknowledge just how important it is to reconnect with yourself and that mindfulness gives you the opportunity to find contentment and calm in the forever changing challenges of motherhood.

Mindfulness is within you if you open yourself up to it, whatever the circumstances it is there to guide you. All we really have is this moment right now – pause, breathe and take it in.

There is always the chance to try again tomorrow. Be kind to yourself, always.

Love Izzy x

Acknowledgements

A huge thank you to everybody at Michael Joseph who has been involved with *Mindfulness for Mums*, particularly Helena Fouracre and Claire Bush in marketing, Olivia Thomas in publicity, Lauren Wakefield in design and my copy-editors, Jennie Roman and Nick Lowndes. It has been wonderful to be surrounded by such a committed and inspiring team.

A special thank you to my editor Charlotte Hardman for giving me confidence, encouragement and for sharing my vision. Thank you for always being at the end of the phone and for your constant support and guidance.

Thank you to my agent Stephanie Thwaites, who continues to help make it possible for me to write about subjects that mean so much to me.

My managers and friends Sophie and Kim at River Talent, thank you for your kindness, dedication and hard work.

Harry, thank you for helping me to keep a sense of humour and perspective, and for giving me the space and time to write. You are the best husband and dad – we love you so much.

Lola and Kit, the heart of this book is inspired by you. Mindfulness is always there within you and I promise to teach you as best I can so that in those challenging moments, mindfulness will be your friend just as it has been mine.

Index

A

accept 77, 79, 81
affirmations 15–17, 89,
    130–31
Anderson, Mac 120
anxiety 2–4
  letting go 83–9
autopilot awareness
    193–5

B

bath time 46
bedtime 91–101, 103–7
  see also sleep

body 30–31
body scan 32–3
  bedtime 94–5
boredom jar 74–6
breathing 42
  bedtime 93–4
  breathing cycle 25–7
  children's exercises
    41–6
  letting go 88
  one-minute
    mindfulness 30–31
  Take five 57–60
bubbles 85–6

C

Calm begins with me
53–6, 130, 162
chakras 143–4, 157–8
crown chakra 156–7
heart chakra 150–51
root chakra 144–5
sacral chakra 146–7
solar plexus chakra
148–9
third-eye chakra 154–5
throat chakra 152–3
children: bedtime 91–101
boredom jar 74–6
breathing exercises
41–6
charge up your hearts
243–5
and emotions 161–9
family list 229–32
gratitude 248, 257–9
jar of hearts 256
letting go 85–7
may you be 103–7
mindfulness 9, 10–11

mindfulness corner
22–3
and nature 171–6
nothing time 73–4
sharing mindful
moments with
213–17
clouds 173
colouring 217–19
comforters 98
crown chakra 156–7

E

emails 184, 186
emotions 162
faces 168–9
guided meditation
164–6
learning about 163–4
letting go 83–9
RAIN 77–82
talking about 167–8
and weather 161–6
extended mountain pose
38–9
eyes: self-care 115

F

face relaxation 116
faces 168–9
family *see* children;
    motherhood
family list 229–32
feeling 31
feelings *see* emotions
5 4 3 2 1 63–6
four sticks 174

G

gardens 176
gift for the day 118
gratitude 247–59
grounding exercise 50–52

H

hands: breathing hands
    45–6
    hand on your heart
    116–18
    holding hands 87
Headspace app 128
hearing 31

heart chakra 150–51
hearts: charge up your
    hearts 243–5
    hand on your heart
    116–18
    holding hands 87
hydration 39, 139–42

I

I spy 173–4
investigate 77, 79, 82

K

Kabat-Zin, Jon 4
kindness 233–41
Knost, L. R. 53

L

Lee, Jennifer Dukes
    233
lemon water 140–42
Lennon, John 71
letters 249–50
letting go 83–9
    charge up your hearts
    243–5

listening 31, 205–9
love wall 214

M

meditation: and chakras
145, 147, 149, 151,
153, 155, 157–8
weather and emotions
164–6
memory book 215–16
mind 30–31
mindfulness 4–5, 9–10,
261–2
affirmation 15–17,
89
autopilot awareness
exercise 194–5
breathing cycle 25–7
breathing exercises
with children 41–6
for children 9, 10–11
finding the time 17–20
kindness exercise
235–6
listening exercise
207–8

mindfulness corner
21–4, 41–2
and motherhood
129–30
and music 220–24
one-minute
mindfulness 29–33
perspective exercise
198–9
reading 225–7
sharing mindful
moments with
family 213–27
slowing down 203–4
and technology 185–7
mobile phones *see* phones
Mother Teresa 259
motherhood 7–9, 11,
121–5, 261–2
early days 129–31
help and support
125–6
multitasking 189–91
and perspective 197–9
relationships 126–7
self-care 111–12

sleep and screens
127–8
starting the day 35–9
well-being 128
mountain pose 38–9
multitasking 189–91
music 119–20, 220–24
playlist 216–17

N

nature 171–6
non-identify 77, 80, 82
nothing time 71–6

O

one-minute mindfulness
29–33, 38, 43, 130

P

phones 128, 179–85
and mindfulness 185–7
photographs: memory
book 215–16
plants 175–6
playlist 216–17

R

RAIN 77–82, 162
rainbow of friendship
98–9
random acts of kindness
238–9
reading 225–7
recognize 77, 78, 81
root chakra 144–5

S

sacral chakra 146–7
screens *see* phones
self-care 1–2, 111–15
chakras 143–58
face relaxation 116
gift for the day 118
going back to
something you
love 118–20
hand on your heart
116–18
motherhood 111–12,
121–31
sleep 133–7

tired eyes 115
water 139–42
singing 220–21
sleep 92, 133–7
    letting go 85
    and motherhood
        127–8
    and screens 127–8,
        184–5
    see also bedtime
'The Sleepy Meadow'
    96–8
slowing down 203–4
snake breathing 44–5
social media 180–81, 183
solar plexus chakra 148–9
sprinkles 100
starting the day 35–9, 141
story time 225–7

T

Take five 57–60
technology 179–87
teddy breathing 44
Tew, Robert 179
THINK 69–70, 162
third-eye chakra 154–5

throat chakra 152–3
Tommy's 125
touch 31

V

visualization: and
        perspective 199
    and sleep 96–8, 136–7

W

WAIT 68–70, 130, 162
wake up with the sun in
        your heart 101
wall of love 214
water 39, 139–42
weather: and emotions
        161–9
Winnie-the-Pooh 213,
        225–6
worry box 86–7

Y

yoga: and chakras 145,
        146, 148, 150, 152,
        154, 156
    extended mountain
        pose 38–9